TELe-Health

Recent advances in technology and medicine are rapidly changing the face of health care. A revolution is occurring in diagnosis and treatment thanks to the implementation of instrumentation and techniques deriving from engineering and research. In addition, a cultural conversion is taking place in which geographical and social boundaries are about to be overcome, resulting in enhanced availability and quality of care. Telemedicine has been considered a possible means of improving health care worldwide that is likely to change the way in which doctors deal with patients and diseases. While various restraints continue to limit the application of telemedicine in different settings and different areas of health, the innovations emerging from eHealth and telecare could stimulate a great leap forward for medicine, provided that some basic rules are taken into consideration and followed. In this series, diverse aspects of tele-health – preventive, promotive, and curative – will be covered by leading experts in the field with the aim of realizing the full potential of the new and exciting technological solutions at our disposal.

Fatih Özden • Zübeyir Sari • Nazan Tuğay
Editors

Telerehabilitation

Springer

Editors
Fatih Özden
Köyceğiz Vocational School of Health Services, Department of Health Care Services
Muğla Sıtkı Koçman University
Muğla, Türkiye

Zübeyir Sari
Faculty of Health Sciences, Department of Physiotherapy and Rehabilitation
Marmara University
Istanbul, Türkiye

Nazan Tuğay
SANKO University, Faculty of Health Sciences, Department of Physiotherapy and Rehabilitation
Gaziantep, Türkiye

ISSN 2198-6037 ISSN 2198-6045 (electronic)
TELe-Health
ISBN 978-3-031-69079-2 ISBN 978-3-031-69080-8 (eBook)
https://doi.org/10.1007/978-3-031-69080-8

This Springer imprint is published by the registered company Springer Nature Switzerland AG
The registered company address is: Gewerbestrasse 11, 6330 Cham, Switzerland

Preface

Telerehabilitation is evolving into a more actively used health service day by day. When remote assessment, treatment, and rehabilitation activities are observed more frequently in practice, telemedicine services that stand out in different rehabilitation disciplines should be considered together with discipline-specific clinical implications. Especially considering the lack of clinical guidelines and ethical principles, it is essential to standardize telerehabilitation services within frameworks in order to provide more efficient health services.

This book is a practical guide for rehabilitation professionals in orthopaedic, neurological, cardiopulmonary, paediatric, and geriatric rehabilitation. It highlights the parameters specific to each field independently by addressing current assessment, physiotherapy, and rehabilitation services independently from each other. In particular, the concepts of teleassessment and telerehabilitation provide solutions to different clinical situations. While remote assessments provide a unique advantage in terms of time and cost, telerehabilitation services can provide an alternative to clinic-based treatment applications when necessary.

Our book addresses telerehabilitation not only in its clinical dimension but also in its legal and ethical dimensions. As in all rehabilitation practices, ethical principles are particularly emphasized in the field of physiotherapy and rehabilitation. Although guidelines have started to be published in recent years, it is seen that the ethical principles and requirements specific to the field are not detailed. It is known that there are different ethical principles, especially for teleassessment and telerehabilitation. By pointing out these problems, our book contains important conclusions that can provide a preliminary source for future telerehabilitation ethical guidelines.

We aim to present the current state of telemedicine-based physiotherapy and rehabilitation services independently and comprehensively, helping stakeholders in the healthcare system make the most of the opportunities in this field. We believe that our book will provide a comprehensive perspective on the revolutionary potential of telemedicine in rehabilitation. We anticipate that academic institutions and healthcare professionals will find this book a helpful tool.

As the editors of this book, which is tailored to physiotherapy and rehabilitation professionals, other healthcare professionals, and academic researchers, we are deeply grateful to all the authors, the editorial team, and the esteemed publishing house. Their collective efforts have been instrumental in bringing this book to fruition, and we extend our heartfelt thanks for their invaluable contributions.

Best regards,

Muğla, Turkey Fatih Özden
Istanbul, Turkey Zübeyir Sarı
Gaziantep, Turkey Nazan Tuğay

Contents

Teleassessment Methods in Orthopedic Rehabilitation

1

Nuray Elibol and Serkan Bakırhan

1.1 Introduction

Assessment has an important place in orthopedic physiotherapy practice to measure the effectiveness of rehabilitation interventions. Assessment includes methods for classifying and measuring a person's variable [1]. In physiotherapy applications, the evaluation of a patient is the basis of treatment. With a good assessment, an effective treatment program can be drawn up [2]. Orthopedic physiotherapy and assessment methods analyze patients' pain, physical function, and exercise control [3]. Teleassessment is the remote assessment of patients within the scope of physiotherapy practice [1–5]. This evaluation method has some advantages. Patients living in rural areas have difficulties and problems reaching the hospital. With teleassessment methods, patients are provided with equal opportunity in treatment [6]. Teleassessment methods such as video and virtual reality can be used, especially in patients who cannot travel long distances due to motor dysfunctions. Considering the problems of access to the clinic due to pain, muscle strength, and joint movement limitations in orthopedic diseases, teleassessment methods come to the fore [7]. These patients must be followed up regularly and timely with routine follow-up and frequent evaluation. In addition, teleassessment methods are becoming important to minimize the risk of transmission due to close contact during the pandemic. Teleassessment methods can also provide an important advantage for patients who cannot receive hospital services due to pain, mobility limitations, and distance to the hospital [8].

Performance-based tests are used in the evaluation of functional outcomes of orthopedic diseases. Physical performance tests emphasize the patient's level of

N. Elibol (✉) · S. Bakırhan
Department of Physiotherapy and Rehabilitation, Faculty of Health Sciences, Ege University, Izmir, Turkey
e-mail: nuray.elibol@ege.edu.tr

F. Özden et al. (eds.), *Telerehabilitation*, TELe-Health,
https://doi.org/10.1007/978-3-031-69080-8_1

competence. These tests are used to indicate changes in functionality. Tests are those in which the patient is assessed by doing the activity himself/herself. These tests include functional and performance tests such as normal range of motion, muscle strength, balance, and gait [9]. However, the difficulties and reliability of teleassessment methods in patients who cannot be evaluated face-to-face due to distance are questioned. Studies have reported that range of motion, muscle strength, balance, gait, and some functional activities can be assessed with teleassessment [3, 10]. However, one of the challenges in integrating teleassessment methods into regular clinical practice is to ensure the validity and reliability of objective assessment methods [2]. In orthopedic diseases, the validity and reliability of teleassessment methods and determining the patient's condition are essential for the clinician to guide the patient correctly and observe recovery. For this reason, the validity and reliability of teleassessment methods have been investigated in many aspects of the literature [10]. The literature reports good concurrent validity between pain, swelling, range of motion, muscle strength, balance, gait, and functional assessments of telerehabilitation evaluations [8, 10]. However, several specialized orthopedic and neurodynamic tests have reported low-to-moderate validity. The diagnostic agreement was assessed compared to face-to-face assessments, and its validity was moderate [11]. Although the level of reliability of teleassessment methods in orthopedic diseases continues to be a subject of research, telehealth studies indicate that these patients have a high level of patient satisfaction. This situation is important in terms of showing the value given to physiotherapy by orthopedic patients who try to access care services through telehealth [12].

In addition to the advantages of teleassessment methods, their use has some disadvantages and limitations. Patients with mental, visual, speech, and hearing problems may not be able to be evaluated by the teleassessment method. In addition, the physiotherapist may need more knowledge and experience in teleassessment. Conducting the assessment online raises concerns about privacy and skepticism among patients. Another limitation or disadvantage is that remote assessment cannot provide the therapeutic effect of touch [1, 6].

The prevalence of the applications in orthopedic diseases in which muscle strength, normal joint movement, posture, pain, and functional levels are evaluated is gradually increasing. Considering the advantages of this situation, it is thought to be promising for physiotherapists.

1.2 Teleassessment Methods

1.2.1 Smartphone-Based Assessments

Mobile applications enable the computerized application of tests in the clinic. Range of motion (ROM) measurement is important in clinical evaluation. For this reason, the need for portable devices has increased for faster and easier applications [13].

Smartphone-based ROM tests have been developed for many joints in the body, and their reliability and validity have been proven. There are also applications for computerized trunk endurance tests [14], exercise capacity tests (e.g., 2- and 6-min walk tests) [15], functional mobility assessment, and gait tests [16] that analyze movement or posture with IMU sensors or a smartphone camera. Wearable devices are also used for movement and posture analysis [17].

Joint range of motion mobile applications: Smartphones can measure joint positions and range of motion statically and dynamically through their gyroscopes, magnetometers, accelerometers, and cameras. Mobile applications that measure joint range of motion can be used on phones and tablets with both IOS and Android operating systems. These applications are as follows [18, 19]:

Muscle strength assessment mobile applications: Manual muscle testing types have been used to evaluate muscle strength for many years. However, there are some limitations in classifying different muscle strengths. Mobile-based applications with gyroscopes, accelerometers, and sensors, along with objective assessment of muscle strength, become part of the self-management strategy for the patient to follow the exercise regime at home and share the digital audit trail of progress with the remote physiotherapist [20].

Posture and anthropometric assessment mobile applications: Posture is the alignment of each body part in the optimal position relative to neighboring parts and the whole body [21, 22]. Correct postural alignment contributes to functions with correct transmission and support [23]. Poor posture paves the way for musculoskeletal disorders such as pain, impaired proprioceptive feedback, muscle activity imbalance, normal joint movement reduction, abnormal load bearing on joints and ligaments, easy fatigue, and increased risk of falling. These changes have a multifactorial etiology and may also be genetic, such as idiopathic scoliosis and hyperkyphosis [24, 25]. Evaluation of postural alignment is one of the most frequently performed evaluations. Due to the important need to identify and manage problems arising from posture disorders, it is used by physiotherapists and other rehabilitation specialists in populations of all ages [23].

Mobile apps use features available on smartphones to assess body alignment and are classified according to these features into sensor-based and image-based measurements. Different types of sensors are used, such as gyroscopes and accelerometers built into smartphones. These sensors capture the displacement or part of the body or are applied to the analysis of radiographic images that provide helpful information about the orientation of spinal segments, including isolated sections (e.g., cervical spine) (Figs. 1.1 and 1.2) [23].

Evaluation of anthropometry can be done both face-to-face and remotely, with high-resolution, depth-of-field cameras, microsensor hardware on smartphones, and software that works integrated with this hardware. These mobile applications are as follows [1]:

Mobile Anthropometry Applications

BodyMeasurement diary

BodyProgress Tracker

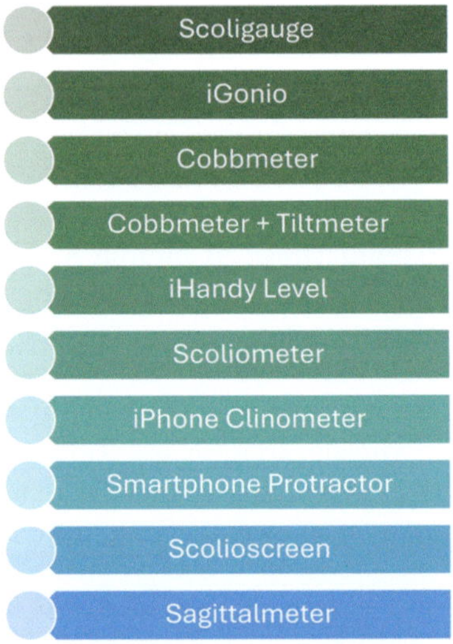

Fig. 1.1 Sensor-based mobile ROM applications

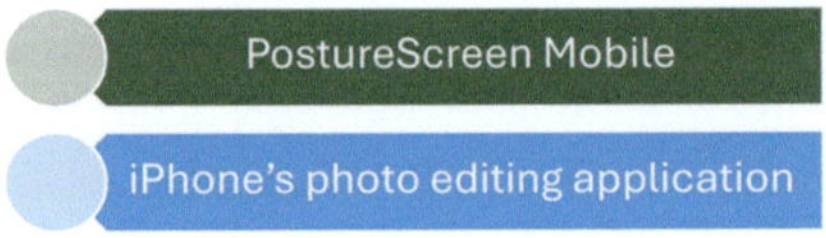

Fig. 1.2 Image-based mobile ROM applications

AntroCal
Body Measurement
Remeasure
Angulus

Physical function and mobility assessment applications: The importance of using technological devices to sustain and monitor rehabilitation programs in patients with musculoskeletal disorders has increased [26]. A standardized assessment of physical function and physical performance also represents an important need in home-based rehabilitation programs to personalize therapeutic intervention and monitor the benefits of the comprehensive rehabilitation program [27]. Innovations in mobile health technology make it easier to evaluate physical function and mobility. Most smartphones can reliably analyze functions such as sit-to-stand, stepping up, and walking with sensors such as accelerometers, gyroscopes, and magnetometers [28, 29]. These applications include self-evaluation of tests such as timed-up and go, sit-to-stand, 10-m walking test, 6-min walking test, etc., which are frequently used in the evaluation of physical function and mobility [28].

Survey/scale applications: Disease-related survey applications frequently used in patient tele-evaluation have both mobile and web-based applications. These applications have begun to be used frequently due to advantages such as their understandability and saving space and time. Some of the mobile questionnaires/scales used to evaluate parameters such as pain, physical performance, mobility, and balance in orthopedic diseases are as follows [30]:

Mobile Survey/Scale Applications
VASQ Clinical
Orebro Musculoskeletal Pain Screening Tool
Musculoskeletal Flag Screening Tool
m-WOMAC
StarTBack Low Back Pain
Berg Balance Scale
Frailty tool
Geriatric
SPPB Calculator
Gait Speed

1.2.2 Videoconferencing-Based Assessment

Physiotherapy assessment using real-time digital technology typically involves audio and visual communication between the patient and the physiotherapist via a videoconferencing system using a computer, tablet, or smartphone [31].

Tele-evaluation via videoconferencing consists of video tests that facilitate specific physical examination techniques that remote and rural patients can perform independently. Many of these tests are based on validated physical examination maneuvers performed during face-to-face patient encounters but have been modified to allow the patient to perform the maneuvers independently. Under the guidance of a remote therapist, the patient must self-examine and self-perform certain functional and orthopedic tests [32, 33].

Joint range of motion assessment via videoconferencing: Joint movement assessment can be done remotely with the sufficient technological infrastructure of a videoconference connection. Videoconference Goniometer® (VG) is a system that provides remote assessment of ROM via videoconferencing. VG® consists of a personal computer, videoconferencing hardware, a video camera with a microphone, a software application, and two interfaces: patient and hospital mode. Patient mode is located in the patient's home and consists of a screen connected to the computer. Hospital mode allows goniometric analysis to be performed on snapshots by capturing movements during live interaction via a videoconference [34].

Suppose the patient has a relative/caregiver with him/her to evaluate ROM with video conference (VC) synchronously. In that case, the physiotherapist instructs the relative/caregiver to place the goniometer on the joint and asks the patient to perform the movement. Then, the physiotherapist zooms in on the camera and reads the value directly, or the patient's relative/caregiver reports the value read on the goniometer to the physiotherapist. In asynchronous evaluation, the physiotherapist asks the patient to move the joint whose ROM will be measured and takes an instant screenshot. The image is then transferred to the virtual goniometer application by the physiotherapist; anatomical points are marked on the patient's image with the cursor, and the angle is automatically calculated [35].

Muscle strength assessment via videoconferencing: Muscle strength can be evaluated using special digital dynamometers, sensors connected to the computer's serial port, and the computer interface unit. When the patient's relative/caregiver applies pressure to the patient's muscle to be evaluated with a dynamometer, the force detected by the sensors is transferred to the computer interface. The patient's muscle strength is assessed based on the muscle strength result data sent to the physiotherapist's computer [1].

Physical function and mobility assessment via videoconferencing: Physical performance tests, an important component of telehealth assessments and exercise programs, provide information about individuals' general health status and quality of life [36]. These tests can be performed 1:1 synchronously via videoconferencing and evaluated with various systems. eHAB is an exemplary computer-based videoconferencing system that enables remote consultations between patients and healthcare professionals via a wireless 3G Internet connection (Telstra Next GÔ; Telstra, Melbourne, VIC, Australia). The system includes measurement tools that objectively measure the participant's physical performance (such as balance and gait assessment) via an Internet connection. This system has features such as real-time videoconferencing, storing and transmitting still images of the participant, and remote camera pan-zoom control [35].

References

1. Köse N, Keser İ, Kayabınar E, Türkmen C. Telerehabilitasyon fizyoterapi uygulamalari. Ankara: Hipokrat Kitabevi; 2022.
2. Durfee WK, Savard L, Weinstein S. Technical feasibility of teleassessments for rehabilitation. IEEE Trans Neural Syst Rehabil Eng. 2007;15(1):23–9. https://doi.org/10.1109/tnsre.2007.891400.
3. Bernhardsson S, Larsson A, Bergenheim A, Ho-Henriksson C-M, Ekhammar A, Lange E, et al. Digital physiotherapy assessment vs conventional face-to-face physiotherapy assessment of patients with musculoskeletal disorders: a systematic review. PLoS One. 2023;18(3):e0283013. https://doi.org/10.1371/journal.pone.0283013.
4. Stephenson A, Howes S, Murphy PJ, Deutsch JE, Stokes M, Pedlow K, et al. Factors influencing the delivery of telerehabilitation for stroke: a systematic review. PLoS One. 2022;17(5):e0265828. https://doi.org/10.1371/journal.pone.0265828.
5. Amin J, Ahmad B, Amin S, Siddiqui AA, Alam MK. Rehabilitation professional and patient satisfaction with telerehabilitation of musculoskeletal disorders: a systematic review. Biomed Res Int. 2022;2022:7366063. https://doi.org/10.1155/2022/7366063.
6. ÖZden F, Arik AF, TuĞAy N. Ortopedik fizyoterapi alaninda güncel telerehabilitasyon yaklaşimlari. Curr Telerehabil Approach Orthop Physiother. 2020;5(2):354–60. https://doi.org/10.5336/healthsci.2019-70990.
7. Hailey D, Roine R, Ohinmaa A, Dennett L. Evidence of benefit from telerehabilitation in routine care: a systematic review. J Telemed Telecare. 2011;17(6):281–7. https://doi.org/10.1258/jtt.2011.101208.
8. Cottrell MA, Russell TG. Telehealth for musculoskeletal physiotherapy. Musculoskelet Sci Pract. 2020;48:102193. https://doi.org/10.1016/j.msksp.2020.102193.
9. Bakirhan S, Angin S, Karatosun V, Unver B, Gunal I. Physical performance parameters during standing up in patients with unilateral and bilateral total knee arthroplasty. Acta Orthop Traumatol Turc. 2012;46(5):367–72.

10. Mani S, Sharma S, Singh DKA. Concurrent validity and reliability of telerehabilitation-based physiotherapy assessment of cervical spine in adults with non-specific neck pain. J Telemed Telecare. 2019;27(2):88–97. https://doi.org/10.1177/1357633X19861802.
11. Çelik EB. Kas iskelet sistemi hastalıklarında telerehabilitasyon. J Med Topics Updates. 2023;2(3):74–80. https://doi.org/10.58651/jomtu.1389337.
12. Lawford BJ, Delany C, Bennell KL, Hinman RS. "I was really sceptical…But it worked really well": a qualitative study of patient perceptions of telephone-delivered exercise therapy by physiotherapists for people with knee osteoarthritis. Osteoarthr Cartil. 2018;26(6):741–50. https://doi.org/10.1016/j.joca.2018.02.909.
13. Cruz J, Morais N. Intrarater agreement of elbow extension range of motion in the upper limb neurodynamic test 1 using a smartphone application. Arch Phys Med Rehabil. 2016;97(11):1880–6. https://doi.org/10.1016/j.apmr.2016.05.001.
14. Banos O, Moral-Munoz JA, Diaz-Reyes I, Arroyo-Morales M, Damas M, Herrera-Viedma E, et al. mDurance: a novel Mobile health system to support trunk endurance assessment. Sensors. 2015;15(6):13159–83. https://doi.org/10.3390/s150613159.
15. Capela NA, Lemaire ED, Baddour N. Feature selection for wearable smartphone-based human activity recognition with able bodied, elderly, and stroke patients. PLoS One. 2015;10(4):e0124414. https://doi.org/10.1371/journal.pone.0124414.
16. Perez AA, Labrador MA. A smartphone-based system for clinical gait assessment. In: 2016 IEEE International Conference on Smart Computing (SMARTCOMP). 2016. p. 1–8.
17. Moral-Munoz PhD JA, Zhang PhD W, Cobo PhD MJ, Herrera-Viedma PhD E, Kaber PhD DB. Smartphone-based systems for physical rehabilitation applications: a systematic review. Assist Technol. 2021;33(4):223–36. https://doi.org/10.1080/10400435.2019.1611676.
18. Milani P, Coccetta CA, Rabini A, Sciarra T, Massazza G, Ferriero G. Mobile smartphone applications for body position measurement in rehabilitation: a review of goniometric tools. PM R. 2014;6(11):1038–43. https://doi.org/10.1016/j.pmrj.2014.05.003.
19. Lau T, Lin S, Wu W, McKivigan JM. Reliability and validity of a smartphone-based inclinometer application measuring shoulder internal rotation. J Phys Fitness Med Treatment Sports. 2020;7(5):e555725.
20. Mukherjee D, Arvind DK. Muscle strength testing using wearable wireless sensors. In: Proceedings of the 10th EAI international conference on body area networks. Sydney: ICST (Institute for Computer Sciences, Social-Informatics and Telecommunications Engineering); 2015. p. 58–61.
21. Claus AP, Hides JA, Moseley GL, Hodges PW. Is 'ideal' sitting posture real?: measurement of spinal curves in four sitting postures. Man Ther. 2009;14(4):404–8. https://doi.org/10.1016/j.math.2008.06.001.
22. Hazar Z, Karabicak GO, Tiftikci U. Reliability of photographic posture analysis of adolescents. J Phys Ther Sci. 2015;27(10):3123–6. https://doi.org/10.1589/jpts.27.3123.
23. Moreira R, Teles A, Fialho R, Baluz R, Santos TC, Goulart-Filho R, et al. Mobile applications for assessing human posture: a systematic literature review. Electronics. 2020;9(8):1196. https://doi.org/10.3390/electronics9081196.
24. Jiang H, Yang F, Lin T, Shao W, Meng Y, Ma J, et al. Asymmetric expression of H19 and ADIPOQ in concave/convex paravertebral muscles is associated with severe adolescent idiopathic scoliosis. Mol Med. 2018;24(1):48. https://doi.org/10.1186/s10020-018-0049-y.
25. Yau MS, Demissie S, Zhou Y, Anderson DE, Lorbergs AL, Kiel DP, et al. Heritability of thoracic spine curvature and genetic correlations with other spine traits: the Framingham study. J Bone Miner Res. 2016;31(12):2077–84. https://doi.org/10.1002/jbmr.2925.
26. Lippi L, Desimoni F, Canonico M, Massocco G, Turco A, Polverelli M, et al. System for tracking and evaluating performance (Step-App®): validation and clinical application of a mobile telemonitoring system in patients with knee and hip total arthroplasty. A prospective cohort study. Eur J Phys Rehabil Med. 2024;60(2):349–60. https://doi.org/10.23736/s1973-9087.24.08128-0.
27. Nilsdotter A-K, Roos EM, Westerlund JP, Roos HP, Lohmander LS. Comparative responsiveness of measures of pain and function after total hip replacement. Arthritis

Care Res. 2001;45(3):258–62. https://doi.org/10.1002/1529-0131(200106)45:3<258::AID-ART258>3.0.CO;2-L.

28. Bergquist R, Vereijken B, Mellone S, Corzani M, Helbostad JL, Taraldsen K. App-based self-administrable clinical tests of physical function: development and usability study. JMIR Mhealth Uhealth. 2020;8(4):e16507. https://doi.org/10.2196/16507.
29. Mellone S, Tacconi C, Chiari L. Validity of a smartphone-based instrumented timed up and go. Gait Posture. 2012;36(1):163–5. https://doi.org/10.1016/j.gaitpost.2012.02.006.
30. Bellamy N, Wilson C, Hendrikz J, Whitehouse SL, Patel B, Dennison S, et al. Osteoarthritis Index delivered by mobile phone (m-WOMAC) is valid, reliable, and responsive. J Clin Epidemiol. 2011;64(2):182–90. https://doi.org/10.1016/j.jclinepi.2010.03.013.
31. Drossman DA, Chang L, Bellamy N, Gallo-Torres HE, Lembo A, Mearin F, et al. Severity in irritable bowel syndrome: a Rome Foundation Working Team Report. Am J Gastroenterol. 2011;106(10):1749–59; quiz 1760.
32. Zischke C, Simas V, Hing W, Milne N, Spittle A, Pope R. The utility of physiotherapy assessments delivered by telehealth: a systematic review. J Glob Health. 2021;11:04072. https://doi.org/10.7189/jogh.11.04072.
33. Grona SL, Bath B, Busch A, Rotter T, Trask C, Harrison E. Use of videoconferencing for physical therapy in people with musculoskeletal conditions: a systematic review. J Telemed Telecare. 2017;24(5):341–55. https://doi.org/10.1177/1357633X17700781.
34. Bernard M-M, Janson F, Flora PK, Faulkner GEJ, Meunier-Norman L, Fruhwirth M. Videoconference-based physiotherapy and tele-assessment for homebound older adults: a pilot study. Act Adapt Aging. 2009;33(1):39–48. https://doi.org/10.1080/01924780902718608.
35. Truter P, Russell T, Fary R. The validity of physical therapy assessment of low back pain via telerehabilitation in a clinical setting. Telemed eHealth. 2013;20(2):161–7. https://doi.org/10.1089/tmj.2013.0088.
36. Espin A, García-García J, Latorre Erezuma U, Aiestaran M, Irazusta J, Rodriguez-Larrad A. Videoconference-based physical performance tests: reliability and feasibility study. Int J Environ Res Public Health. 2022;19(12):7109. https://doi.org/10.3390/ijerph19127109.

2 Telerehabilitation Methods in Orthopedic Rehabilitation

İsmet Tümtürk and Serkan Bakırhan

2.1 Introduction

Orthopedic diseases include inflammatory and degenerative conditions affecting muscles, tendons, ligaments, nerves, bones, and joints. It is one of the significant public health problems whose prevalence is increasing worldwide [1]. According to the World Health Organization, diseases such as osteoarthritis, osteoporosis, fractures, rheumatoid arthritis, and waist and neck pain are among the most common orthopedic diseases. Low back pain, which is the most critical disorder affecting the musculoskeletal system, has been listed among the problems that cause the most disability since 1990 [2, 3]. About two and a half billion people worldwide need rehabilitation due to various illnesses. This number is gradually increasing. Orthopedic rehabilitation has a vital role in restoring impaired function after trauma or surgery. The increase in the elderly population worldwide and changes in population needs have made it necessary to develop new rehabilitation models and practices [4]. Exercise practices under the supervision of a physiotherapist are essential. However, the development of new information technologies and telemedical devices has made telerehabilitation practices widespread in recent years. The decrease in Internet costs has increased the opportunity to apply technology-based solutions to maintain health services inside and outside the hospital [5, 6]. Telerehabilitation

İ. Tümtürk
Department of Physiotherapy and Rehabilitation, Institute of Health Sciences, Süleyman Demirel University, Isparta, Turkey

Department of Physiotherapy and Rehabilitation, Faculty of Health Sciences, Antalya Bilim University, Antalya, Turkey

S. Bakırhan (✉)
Department of Physiotherapy and Rehabilitation, Faculty of Health Sciences, Ege University, İzmir, Turkey
e-mail: serkan.bakirhan@ege.edu.tr

F. Özden et al. (eds.), *Telerehabilitation*, TELe-Health,
https://doi.org/10.1007/978-3-031-69080-8_2

provides remote rehabilitation services through technological methods such as videos, telephone, videoconferencing platforms, or virtual reality [7]. In recent years, it has been widely used in the implementation of evaluation and treatment programs in neurological, pulmonary, geriatric, and pediatric patients, primarily orthopedic diseases [8].

Studies have shown that telerehabilitation applications are a feasible and effective method for many diseases, especially orthopedic diseases [9, 10]. In recent years, the need for telerehabilitation has increased to reduce physical density in hospitals, to provide rapid access to patients waiting for rehabilitation services, and to effectively continue the treatment of patients who are difficult to transfer to the hospital. Technology-based rehabilitation services have emerged as a promising alternative method, especially in the postsurgical period. With the COVID-19 pandemic, telerehabilitation practices have come to the fore to reduce physical contact and protect the health of patients and physiotherapists [11, 12]. In cases where digital services cannot be provided in sufficient quantities, especially in rural areas, telerehabilitation applications are essential in eliminating health service inequality in orthopedic diseases [13]. Telerehabilitation practices are alternative practices to traditional and face-to-face treatment methods. It is rapidly becoming widespread in orthopedics because it is a low-cost physiotherapy option. This rehabilitation option includes various services such as education, counseling, supervision, and exercise control [14]. Telerehabilitation applications aim to monitor treatment results, control treatment, and reduce treatment costs.

Many telemedicine methods have been developed in health services, including telenursing, telerehabilitation, teleradiology, and telecardiology. One of these methods is the tele-orthopedics method used to follow up orthopedic diseases [15]. This method is widely used in patients with musculoskeletal disorders in the USA [16]. Tele-orthopedics is one method used via web and telecommunication that does not involve transferring the patient to the hospital or taking up too much time. A total of 88% of this method comprises telemonitoring, and 12% includes telesurgery [17]. Telerehabilitation methods are used in the rehabilitation of orthopedic and musculoskeletal diseases. When current developments are examined, it is seen that clinicians are turning to telerehabilitation-based applications with the latest developments in computer software, biosensors, and communication technology [13]. Technology-based methods are frequently used to evaluate and treat orthopedic-related pathologies in physiotherapy. Orthopedic problems arising from the aging population have led to a greater tendency towards telerehabilitation practices in this field. Recent studies in orthopedic and musculoskeletal rehabilitation show that telerehabilitation practices are practical and sufficient compared to conventional treatment methods [10, 13]. The importance of telerehabilitation emerges in in-hospital and acute rehabilitation interventions and remote monitoring of individuals with chronic health problems. It has been reported that some applications using telephone or videoconferencing effectively overcome the limitations in access to treatment for orthopedic diseases [10]. Telerehabilitation studies in physiotherapy for the musculoskeletal system universally report high levels of patient satisfaction [17].

Research on telerehabilitation applications in musculoskeletal system diseases is rapidly increasing in the literature. Systematic reviews have shown that telehealth can provide health improvements. It is stated that it can effectively reduce pain and functional limitations in cases such as osteoarthritis, low back pain, neck pain, and arthroplasty surgery [10, 18, 19]. Telerehabilitation has also been shown to increase exercise compliance in various musculoskeletal disorders. Significantly, during COVID-19, healthcare institutions have accelerated access to these applications to adopt telehealth quickly. Telerehabilitation practices in musculoskeletal diseases are a feasible and effective alternative for people who cannot access face-to-face healthcare. Although telehabilitation applications in orthopedics will close the gap in access to healthcare services, they are expected to leave a lasting and positive impact on how healthcare services are accessed after COVID-19 [20]. Although telerehabilitation practices are a new application area, they have some areas for improvement and limitations. Besides technological restrictions and usage, patients have some negativities, such as individual reluctance and skepticism. Another limitation is the existence of regulations that financially limit patients' access to telerehabilitation [21]. Despite these factors, telerehabilitation practices continue to develop in orthopedic rehabilitation [22].

Today, telerehabilitation applications are used in many areas, such as hip and knee osteoarthritis, fractures, subacromial impingement syndrome, lower and upper extremity injuries, and presurgical and postsurgical periods.

2.2 Telerehabilitation in Orthopedic Conditions

Synchronous and asynchronous methods can perform telerehabilitation. The synchronous telerehabilitation method uses videoconferencing technologies and requires patients to participate in exercise sessions simultaneously under supervision. Asynchronous telerehabilitation allows patients to access exercise programs using technology devices at their preferred time. Synchronous telerehabilitation helps build the patient-therapist relationship through real-time interaction and increases session access and adherence. However, it requires the simultaneous presence of both patient and therapist, which increases the workload compared to asynchronous telerehabilitation. The program flexibility of asynchronous telerehabilitation reduces the therapist's workload. However, asynchronous telerehabilitation needs more patient-therapist interaction.

Synchronized teleconferencing is when the patient can receive feedback "face-to-face" with the therapist despite being in different locations. This method assists the patient in learning and practicing therapeutic exercises. This live teleconference allows therapists to measure joint angles with an Internet-based goniometer. An added benefit of this remote rehabilitation is that therapists can use motion analysis tools to capture video sequences from the live teleconference. Therapists may explain the importance of physiotherapy, educate patients and caregivers, review exercise programs, and provide real-time coaching, just as in traditional therapy [23].

Asynchronous telerehabilitation consists of recorded videos sent between practitioner and patient. Following a teleconference assessment, recorded videos demonstrating the correct execution of specific exercises can be provided to patients. The patient can provide the therapist with video recordings of their practiced exercises to get feedback. Alternatively, patients can learn therapeutic exercises by watching three-dimensional avatars instead of videos sent by physiotherapists. Patients can perform these exercises by wearing sensors so that their movement trajectories may be analyzed. The therapist can monitor these measurements. This biometric data can be utilized to determine optimal rehabilitation. Through custom programming, the software can also detect when an exercise is being performed inappropriately, alert the therapist, and provide an avatar to guide the patient. Text messages can also provide education, reminders, and encouragement [23, 24].

Website-based telerehabilitation is less similar to traditional therapy than synchronous or asynchronous therapy. However, website-based telerehabilitation can be advantageous for providing therapeutic exercises or information about the disease. Patients always have access to education, exercise logs, medication logs, bulletin boards, and exercise programs. Due to the possibilities of website formatting, the website can be formatted to meet the needs of patients [23].

Through telerehabilitation technologies, therapists also can treat patients individually or in groups. Group sessions involve one therapist providing therapy simultaneously to multiple people in different locations. With the appropriate setup (enough space, Internet, screen, audio, and software), patients can participate in group therapy sessions regardless of the therapist's location. Group sessions connecting virtually with patients have the added benefit of reducing social isolation and using social support to accelerate their recovery. These group sessions can also be enhanced using text messages, sensors, virtual reality avatars, and wearable devices [23]. Another way of developing telerehabilitation technologies is the sensory method used [25].

One of the exciting new areas in telerehabilitation methods is virtual reality. Virtual reality allows the visual, auditory, tactile, and even olfactory senses to be presented to the patient as a representation of the physical experience [26]. In addition, haptic systems that incorporate haptic information in applications, called force feedback, have been developed. Haptic technology interfaces with the patient through the sense of touch by applying force, vibration, or movement. This allows for enhanced adaptation to the virtual environment. This technology provides objective feedback. Another advantage of virtual reality is the protection from the risks of performing the same task in a realistic and dangerous environment. The virtual reality method enhances reality by providing patients with a clinical environment. In addition, the virtual environment is adapted to the patient's condition, and the challenge of the environment is optimized [27, 28]. Management of patients with physical and orthopedic disabilities is provided through multimedia and exergaming techniques. Examples are systems such as "Kinect," "Nintendo Wii," or "Rehab@ Home," which create a virtual environment for the patient [29].

The effects of telerehabilitation have been investigated in a variety of musculoskeletal conditions, including low back pain, lumbar stenosis, osteoarthritis, and neck pain. Benefits include reduced hospitalization, shorter rehabilitation unit stays, reduced burden of accessing outpatient physical therapy, improved quality of life, health outcomes, and early return to work [25]. Telerehabilitation methods are also applied after surgery for orthopedic problems. These interventions include home exercises, communication in addition to home healthcare, telephonic information and support, outpatient rehabilitation with telemedical monitoring, wireless-monitored home-based exercise training, interactive virtual telerehabilitation, telerehabilitation with videoconferencing, electronic health information support, telephonic social support and education, telephone-based physical activity exercise, e-health program [9]. Patient satisfaction is at the forefront of health services. In telerehabilitation, similar to traditional face-to-face meetings, the physiotherapist pays one-to-one attention to the patient and offers personalized therapies. There have been studies showing satisfaction with telerehabilitation, which have demonstrated an overall high degree of satisfaction [30–35].

When choosing a particular telehabilitation technology, it is beneficial for the clinician to consider several factors. Usability is essential as the required technology needs to be accessible to all participants. As patient data requires confidentiality, security must be addressed. Regarding platform security, end-to-end encryption is a requirement [25]. Telerehabilitation has some limitations as well as areas of application. Besides the cost concerns of telerehabilitation, more person-to-person contact is needed to maintain the effectiveness of telerehabilitation. Physiotherapy sessions in the patient's home are contextually different from the clinical setting. In addition, the patient may face equipment barriers, such as the need for weights and bands available in the clinic in the home environment. Patients may also need more technology or knowledge to perform telerehabilitation. Patients should receive adequate education and information before starting treatment. Older adults may have difficulty using telerehabilitation systems. For example, long session duration (recommended not to exceed 30 min) is a factor that can affect dizziness and nausea. Given the barriers listed above, telerehabilitation is an approach that can be used in addition to face-to-face interventions, increasing treatment effectiveness [36–39]. The following discussion of telerehabilitation applications in orthopedic problems will help clinicians to choose appropriate telerehabilitation methods.

2.2.1 Telerehabilitation for Neck Pain

Neck pain is a common condition affecting a significant proportion of the global population [40]. Neck pain increases in cases such as poor posture and excessive phone use. This condition, which causes bad posture, has started to affect the entire population in recent years [41]. This is why it is crucial for patients suffering from neck pain to practice telerehabilitation, which consistently encourages correct posture. Exercise therapy with telerehabilitation can improve outcomes of chronic non-specific neck pain. Improvements are significant when the exercises given for neck pain are monitored frequently with methods such as teleconferencing and text messaging [42].

Exercise therapy is an essential component of rehabilitation for nonspecific neck pain. However, individuals with neck pain often fail to meet exercise guidelines. Telerehabilitation is thought to increase adherence and have positive long-term effects [43]. A study comparing telerehabilitation with face-to-face rehabilitation for neck pain found similar positive effects [44] in another three-group study. An interactive telerehabilitation program (strengthening, motor control, and posture correction exercises), a home exercise program performed by patients on their own, and office ergonomics training alone were compared. The office ergonomics plus interactive telerehabilitation group was the most effective [45]. The usability of the video exercise protocol offered by telerehabilitation was higher than that of conventional methods. Patients' satisfaction and exercise adherence were also higher with telerehabilitation [30]. The effectiveness of synchronous and asynchronous telerehabilitation in individuals with neck pain was also evaluated. Synchronous and asynchronous telerehabilitation were shown to produce similar results. Well-designed asynchronous telerehabilitation methods, that is, asynchronous telerehabilitation methods that include easy-to-use exercise descriptions that are understandable by the patient, can show the same results with less effort without the need for synchronous methods [46].

According to a systematic review meta-analysis, virtual reality may be an effective treatment for neck pain [47]. According to another review, there is moderate quality evidence that virtual reality is an impactful approach [48]. The good news is that for people with neck pain, a head-mounted display does not change neck posture for the worse [40]. There are also website-based guidelines for neck pain from various associations and field authorities. Patients can be guided on how to manage neck pain [49].

All these telerehabilitation applications used in neck pain included deep neck flexor strengthening exercises, facilitation of correct posture, stretching exercises, motor control exercises, stimulation of neck joint movements, stabilization exercises, activities of daily living training, proprioceptive exercises, and McKenzie exercise interventions. Among the telerehabilitation methods applied, synchronous telerehabilitation, asynchronous telerehabilitation, website-based telerehabilitation, and virtual reality can be listed as a combination of various telerehabilitation methods. However, the number of studies conducted using telerehabilitation methods for neck pain is small, and there is a need for more high-quality studies using advanced technologies.

2.2.2 Telerehabilitation for Low Back Pain

Interventions for individuals with nonspecific chronic low back pain include Pilates, stabilization/motor control, resistance training, and aerobic exercise training. In addition, manual therapy and therapist supervision increase the positive effect of treatment [50]. Patients undergoing spine surgery face accessibility concerns that existed before the COVID-19 pandemic and will continue to be a factor to consider in the post-COVID-19 era. The advantages of telerehabilitation are the ability to overcome physical barriers, transportation concerns, and financial limitations [25].

An essential point in telerehabilitation is the ability to visually provide ambient input feedback to patients. A recent study provided participants with low back pain with visual feedback at measurement points on the improvement of outcome measures after practicing home-based exercises with telerehabilitation. As a result, the patients' visual input of the change in their condition contributed more to the improvement [31]. The same logic is present in virtual reality exergame methods. Appropriate clinical environments or targets are visualized and presented to the patient [51–55]. The McKenzie exercise protocol, commonly used in low back pain rehabilitation, can be applied with telerehabilitation, and the results showed similar results when compared to the clinical setting [56–58].

Moreover, exercise and education-based telerehabilitation intervention was as effective as clinical practice regarding pain function [59, 60]. Similarly, neuroscience education, pain education, desensitization, relaxation, pelvic floor stabilization, range of motion, and strengthening exercises were applied through telerehabilitation, and improvement was found [61, 62]. Another study compared the effectiveness of home exercises given with telerehabilitation and home exercises given with paper in low back pain. Telerehabilitation significantly improved pain function, quality of life, and kinesiophobia satisfaction motivation parameters [63].

Machine learning is a promising tool for personalized rehabilitation. Machine learning applied to support clinical decisions has been investigated in low back pain. Machine learning had better results than traditional approaches. Therefore, machine learning is a valuable tool for the future of low back pain rehabilitation and integration into rehabilitation systems [64]. Machine learning can help support clinicians' decisions or guide patients through a personalized treatment plan.

Smartphone applications play an active role in the self-management of low back pain. Moderate-to-good quality evidence has been shown for its effectiveness in low back pain [65]. In addition, website-based telehealth models such as YouTube are available, but some content is reported to be of inadequate quality for low back pain [66]. Telerehabilitation interventions have proven to be beneficial in reducing pain levels in patients with low back pain and sustaining this improvement through

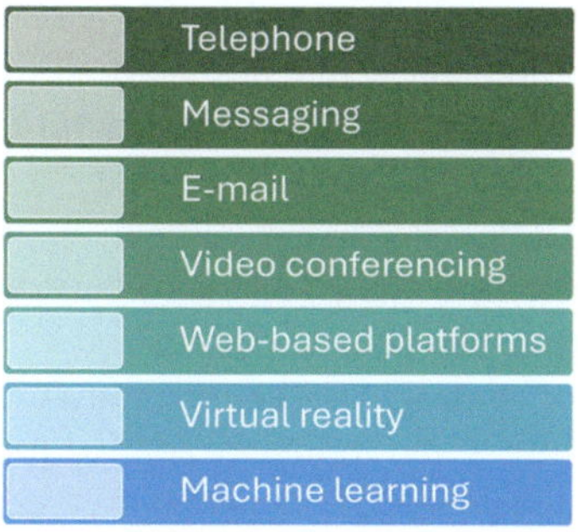

Fig. 2.1 Multimodal systems for telerehabilitation

telerehabilitation. Telerehabilitation methods include multimodal systems such as telephone, messaging, e-mail, videoconferencing, web-based platforms, virtual reality, and machine learning (Fig. 2.1).

2.2.3 Telerehabilitation in Scoliosis

Posture disorders disrupt the daily lives of a significant proportion of the population. Adolescents may also develop scoliosis. In addition, exercise capacity may be reduced even in patients with mild scoliosis [67]. Telerehabilitation contributes to the adherence of individuals with scoliosis to treatment and enables them to perform exercises in the correct pattern. Telerehabilitation has an audiovisual guiding feature. In addition, patients can always access media content. The telerehabilitation program also educates patients and their relatives [68].

Posture-correcting exercises were given in a virtual reality study on adolescents with scoliosis. As a result, it was reported that virtual reality and technological rehabilitation can be practiced for scoliosis [67]. This study was conducted face-to-face, but thanks to the widespread use of virtual reality systems, it can also be applied with the telerehabilitation method in the home environment. Smartphones have accelerometer and gyroscope sensors that enable information to be recorded. Smartphone applications may be beneficial in terms of continuous and easy monitoring and tracking of scoliosis. Through an app, patients' scoliosis measurements and other information are accessed. Thus, telerehabilitation can be utilized to send the patient the exercise prescription that needs to be done now, monitor the effectiveness of the treatment, give instant feedback to the patient without waiting for the clinic visit, and send appointment reminders to the patient [69]. Systems such as Scoliosis Manager, ScolioTrack, Scoliometer, Artificial Intelligence Posture Evaluation, and Correction System can perform accurate evaluations and rehabilitation plans with the support of artificial intelligence by referring to the body protrusions of patients with the help of camera sensors [70]. In addition, the progression of corrective exercises in scoliosis with machine learning provided additional benefits [71].

According to a study applying 3D Schroth treatment, an essential method in treating scoliosis, with teletherapy, telerehabilitation was reported to be a suitable option for exercises that can only be done at home. The face-to-face group improved better than the telerehabilitation group [72]. Another critical approach for individuals with idiopathic scoliosis includes Pilates-based exercises. A study comparing telerehabilitation and home Pilates exercises found that telerehabilitation led to better improvement [73]. In another study, telerehabilitation method was applied to both groups. However, one group received a synchronous method and the other an asynchronous method; which of the two methods was better needed to be clarified. The choice of method must be determined by individual preference from a biopsychological point of view [74]. Telerehabilitation-based spine exoskeleton robots that measure the forces and moments applied to the body, control the direction of body movements, and enable 3D dynamic treatment of scoliosis have also been used [75].

In scoliosis, telerehabilitation applications are a reasonable option to support decreased exercise capacity, teach exercises, provide information about the disease, and follow-up. However, it may be different from conceptual treatments applied face-to-face. It is effective as a supportive treatment.

2.2.4 Telerehabilitation for Shoulder Problems

Shoulder lesions are among the most commonly diagnosed conditions [76]. One of the treatments prescribed in shoulder rehabilitation is exercise-based exercise programs. However, many patients perform their physiotherapeutic exercises incorrectly or less often than prescribed. Telerehabilitation contributes to support exercises done at home.

AGT-Reha, a telerehabilitation system for shoulder rehabilitation, provides real-time feedback. It guides patients through physiotherapeutic exercises at home with automatic real-time feedback. The physiotherapist can remotely observe the quality of home exercises. Physiotherapists can use it to change the number of sets and repetitions per exercise and adjust the difficulty level. AGT-Reha provides participants with an avatar. The findings show that home-based training with AGT-Reha is feasible [76]. Recent research has shown that depth cameras such as Microsoft Kinect, Intel RealSense, and Orbecc are promising for physical function assessment and rehabilitation [77]. The researchers emphasized that telerehabilitation based on machine learning with phone sensors in the frozen shoulder is essential for monitoring patient progress and effective treatment [78]. Primary therapeutic interventions such as warming up, stretching, pain control, range of motion, and muscle strengthening after proximal humerus fracture could be given effectively with telerehabilitation [79]. Another telerehabilitation method was the management of shoulder problems with wearable devices. These devices created an avatar of the person and provided feedback to the patient. The study documented positive results [80]. A hybrid telerehabilitation model (in-clinic and virtual teleconference sessions) was applied in shoulder and thumb arthroplasty patients. As a result, it was found effective in terms of patient satisfaction and upper extremity recovery [81]. Interactive video-based physiotherapy programs at home for patients after shoulder joint replacement showed that they felt safe, competent, and empowered. Access to frequent support, access to feedback, continuity, enhanced communication, specific body knowledge, and being at home contribute to increased recovery competence [82]. A telerehabilitation program including range of motion, rotator cuff strengthening, and scapular stabilizers exercises after shoulder arthroscopy for shoulder impingement syndrome appears to be similar to and not inferior to face-to-face physiotherapy [83]. In other shoulder problems, telerehabilitation also plays an important role [84–86].

A systematic review shows low evidence of no difference between telerehabilitation and home exercise programs. Telerehabilitation is shown to be superior to recommendations to improve shoulder pain disability alone with low evidence [87]. Telerehabilitation interventions included teleconference meetings, progression of exercises by live video call with the patient, the inertial sensor used under the remote supervision of the therapist, presenting exercise videos to patients, transmitting images and protocol via a web platform, teaching self-massage and skin care. Due to the nature of telerehabilitation, manual therapy interventions that cannot be applied to telerehabilitation methods are essential for shoulder problems. Therefore, clinician-based approaches should be considered in addition to telerehabilitation methods for shoulder problems.

2.2.5 Hand Wrist Problems

Hand injuries and hand-related disabilities are common and significant in terms of functional loss and cost [88]. Additional devices often support hand rehabilitation. Devices equipped with electromyography sensors support active movement by measuring the patient's force. Special telemanipulators can also be used for hand telerehabilitation during treatment. The rehabilitation specialist uses the host device to control the patient's hand-mounted device. The rehabilitation process becomes more engaging and motivating when virtual or augmented reality is used [89]. Patients can perform specific exercises guided by photographs prepared by clinicians. The patient is at home, the computer and Internet are available, and the camera is placed on the patient's hand.

The clinician first demonstrates the required hand position. The patient tries to adjust their fingers and wrist accordingly. If the clinician confirms that the patient has performed the task correctly, a photo can be taken and uploaded to the telerehabilitation system. The photo serves as a template for the rehabilitation process. The software installed on the patient's computer automatically downloads the picture and processes the image to contour the hand. At this stage, the patient performs the same exercise, controlling and monitoring their movements through the program. If the program detects the exercise correctly, it informs the patient and moves on to the next task [89]. With the help of artificial intelligence, additional support on the correct exercise pattern can be provided. By integrating AI into VRehab platforms, patients can be offered personalized and outpatient rehabilitation services at home. AI algorithms can make personalized and real-time inferences about the rehabilitation process of patients based on data collected from various sensors [90].

In one study, prescribing telerehabilitation (ReHand) to patients with traumatic bone and soft tissue injuries to the hand, wrist, and fingers improves their functional abilities and reduces the number of face-to-face physiotherapy sessions [88]. With the developing technology, smart, robotic, virtual gloves equipped with sensors can provide exercise assistance according to the correct movement patterns in hand movements [91–94]. Smart gloves can act as an appropriate splint and provide synchronous telerehabilitation and exercise progression by paying attention to the angles of the treatment protocol, which may offer positive effects. Glove systems can also be used in hand replacements [95]. In addition, exercise plus pain neuroscience training increased the effectiveness of telerehabilitation in carpal tunnel syndrome [96]. Telerehabilitation interventions for wrist fractures are performed with tablet-assisted gaming exercises, and wearable exercise aids with sensors that provide feedback. The results showed that telerehabilitation was adequate [97–99]. In contrast, telerehabilitation did not improve exercise adherence, self-efficacy, or range of motion compared to standard rehabilitation in patients followed by mobile application after flexor tendon injury [100].

Telerehabilitation applications for hand rehabilitation are supportive and promising. It can provide joint movements to prevent early adhesions. With telerehabilitation methods, education can be provided to patients and their relatives about complex structures such as the hand. Further developments will be inevitable in a developing and changing world. At the end of the current chapter, the future predictions of the authors are included.

2.2.6 Telerehabilitation for Hip Problems

Orthopedic problems such as hip arthroplasty, hip joint calcification, and hip fractures are frequently encountered, especially in the aging population [101]. Adherence to exercises is essential in these patients. Thanks to the advantages of the telerehabilitation method, specific exercises can be easily implemented. Kinect Rehabilitation System (KiReS), a Kinect-based telerehabilitation system, has been implemented in the literature. This system allows physiotherapists to define exercises by recording themselves with the Kinect's camera. Physiotherapists can thus define a variety of exercises that can be applied to many different health conditions. KiReS offers 3D avatars where patients can observe the movements of their avatars and receive feedback. Patients are supervised by the physiotherapist while performing the exercises, and all the data obtained is recorded in the database [101]. As a result, telerehabilitation was effective with this system [102]. However, this study did not compare telerehabilitation with face-to-face treatment. In a study comparing telerehabilitation (Wellpepper and eHAB) with face-to-face treatment, telerehabilitation was similar to face-to-face training [103]. So, this was an important finding. In a cost study, telerehabilitation was the same as face-to-face care. However, telerehabilitation significantly reduced the time burden for patients and caregivers [104]. Patients liked the convenience of the telerehabilitation program, and surgeons and physiotherapists were satisfied with the protocol [105]. In another study, exercises were sent to patients in video format, and video calls were initiated. In addition, patients were monitored using an electronic thermometer, electronic blood pressure meter, electronic blood glucose meter, and electronic blood oxygen meter that could be connected to the device and transmit the data to the other party. In the other group, the exercises were given in written format, and phone calls were followed. In conclusion, telerehabilitation was effective in health improvements, psychological aspects, and prevention of complications [106, 107].

According to a review focusing on telerehabilitation methods in hip fracture patients, the results of telerehabilitation could have been more precise. It may be necessary to consider telerehabilitation after hip fracture surgery to increase patients' confidence in their ability to perform daily activities without falling [108]. In a review of total hip arthroplasty studies, telerehabilitation interventions showed similar effects to other interventions [109]. Another review reported the benefit of combining telerehabilitation with conventional intervention [110]. In addition, offloading protocols can be implemented via videoconferencing. Moderate- to low-quality evidence of telerehabilitation was presented [111].

2.2.7 Telerehabilitation for Knee Problems

Knee problems are very frequently encountered among orthopedic disorders. Telerehabilitation approaches have also been widely researched in knee problems. In particular, the delivery of home-based exercises and educational content through telerehabilitation methods is effective compared to interventions delivered in a written format [32]. SKYRE, a new platform for remote patient assessment, is used in knee rehabilitation. The platform is based on a multi-sensor wearable garment that can provide real-time objective assessment of physical exercises. This increases patients' awareness and compliance. SKYRE can, therefore, represent a valid alternative for patients and clinicians who wish to conduct an objective assessment and rehabilitation remotely after knee surgery [112]. For a successful recovery after total knee arthroplasty, it is crucial to ensure that rehabilitation is continued at home. Another telerehabilitation system used is ReHub®, which includes an accelerometer, gyroscope, and strain gauge sensors. ReHub®'s algorithms provide real-time biofeedback through an animated talking coach to suggest corrections and motivate the patient.

In conclusion, telerehabilitation with ReHub® is a safe and effective system within the Fast-Track program after hospital discharge [113]. In addition, virtual reality methods are also employed [114]. According to a summary review, videoconferencing-based programs can be considered an alternative to the conventional rehabilitation program for the target group. Recent studies have confirmed the effectiveness of this approach. However, sensor-based solutions may offer higher flexibility and better resource management [115]. Finally, an umbrella review showed that telerehabilitation positively affected walking ability, knee extension, and costs. Regarding quality of life, Western Ontario and McMaster Universities Osteoarthritis Index scores, and patient satisfaction, telerehabilitation had similar effects to conventional rehabilitation [116].

2.2.8 Telerehabilitation for Foot and Ankle Problems

Ankle injuries are among the most common injuries in sports and daily life. Telemedicine literature on foot and ankle-specific applications is even rarer. Problems such as ankle sprains also involve the younger population. This increases the ease of application of telerehabilitation. In addition, foot-related problems limit ambulation, and the advantage of home treatment provided by telerehabilitation may be necessary for these patients. Robots can play an essential role in improving the rehabilitation process.

For this reason, many robotic solutions have been proposed by researchers for upper-limb and lower-limb rehabilitation. Active ankle exercises can be assessed and monitored using wearable motion sensors. In one study, an ankle rehabilitation robot was developed. The ankle robot was intended to be used for telerehabilitation. Visual haptic interfaces were designed to make the exercises engaging and motivating. A library of interactive virtual reality exercises was created to perform a range of motion, muscle strengthening, and balance improvement therapy [116]. Another study used a telewobble board. An accelerometer was installed to detect the tilt angles of the board, which in turn detected the user's ankle tilt. In addition, four vibration motors were mounted on the back of the board to produce vibratory feedback when an exercise was achieved. The system allows the clinician to monitor the patient's progress by reviewing performance parameters remotely [117]. Such balance boards can also be used as a telerehabilitation method in home environments by integrating them with virtual reality or games for lower extremity problems [118–120]. The overall average satisfaction of telemedicine visits for foot and ankle problems was significantly lower than in-office visits. However, patients reported that they would use telemedicine again in the future. Patients who experienced trauma and had more significant barriers to foot and ankle care were more satisfied with telemedicine visits [121]. A study of telerehabilitation for ankle sprains (SWORD Health) achieved clinical outcomes comparable to face-to-face interventions [122]. According to a study investigating the effectiveness of telerehabilitation (web-based and smartphone-enabled) for a hindfoot pain exercise program, the combined systems had a better effect [123].

2.2.9 Telerehabilitation in Chronic Pain

Yoga is a popular form of complementary and integrative medicine that supplements standard medical treatment, and studies provide evidence that yoga practiced via telehealth provides satisfaction and health improvement comparable to in-person yoga [124]. In amputees or chronic pain, such relaxation techniques, understanding chronic pain, pain mechanism, coping with chronic pain, stimulating painless activities, and reducing chronic pain, desensitization can be used more effectively with telerehabilitation systems. Virtual reality and visualization of metaphors are significant in pain management [125, 126].

2.3 Conclusion

Existing telerehabilitation methods can be optimally combined with other treatment modalities according to the person's current level of disability. Telerehabilitation still needs to be superior to face-to-face interventions (manual therapy, etc.). In the future, with the development of technology and communication systems, humanoid artificial intelligence robots that meet all assessment and treatment requirements, such as touch (e.g., end-feel), smell, and tele-radiography, will enter our lives. For example, imagine that the physiotherapist performs manual therapy sessions remotely with the help of a robot. In this way, health professionals will remotely examine and rehabilitate the patient as if they were in a clinical environment, and all the while, they will not lack any senses and requirements.

References

1. Telfer S, Obradovich N. Local weather is associated with rates of online searches for musculoskeletal pain symptoms. PLoS One. 2017;12(8):e0181266. https://doi.org/10.1371/journal.pone.0181266.
2. Behmanesh A, Sadoughi F, Mazhar FN, Joghataei MT, Yazdani S. Tele-orthopaedics: a systematic mapping study. J Telemed Telecare. 2020;28(1):3–23. https://doi.org/10.1177/1357633X20919308.
3. Sebbag E, Felten R, Sagez F, Sibilia J, Devilliers H, Arnaud L. The worldwide burden of musculoskeletal diseases: a systematic analysis of the World Health Organization Burden of Diseases Database. Ann Rheum Dis. 2019;78(6):844–8. https://doi.org/10.1136/annrheumdis-2019-215142.
4. Rogante M, Grigioni M, Cordella D, Giacomozzi C. Ten years of telerehabilitation: a literature overview of technologies and clinical applications. NeuroRehabilitation. 2010;27:287–304. https://doi.org/10.3233/NRE-2010-0612.
5. Agostini M, Moja L, Banzi R, Pistotti V, Tonin P, Venneri A, et al. Telerehabilitation and recovery of motor function: a systematic review and meta-analysis. J Telemed Telecare. 2015;21(4):202–13. https://doi.org/10.1177/1357633X15572201.
6. Rogante M, Kairy D, Giacomozzi C, Grigioni M. A quality assessment of systematic reviews on telerehabilitation: what does the evidence tell us? Ann Ist Super Sanita. 2015;51(1):11–8. https://doi.org/10.4415/ann_15_01_04.
7. Bernhardsson S, Larsson A, Bergenheim A, Ho-Henriksson C-M, Ekhammar A, Lange E, et al. Digital physiotherapy assessment vs conventional face-to-face physiotherapy assessment of patients with musculoskeletal disorders: a systematic review. PLoS One. 2023;18(3):e0283013. https://doi.org/10.1371/journal.pone.0283013.
8. Oh-Park M, Lew HL, Raghavan P. Telerehabilitation for geriatrics. Phys Med Rehabil Clin. 2021;32(2):291–305. https://doi.org/10.1016/j.pmr.2021.01.003.
9. van Egmond MA, van der Schaaf M, Vredeveld T, Vollenbroek-Hutten MMR, van Berge Henegouwen MI, Klinkenbijl JHG, et al. Effectiveness of physiotherapy with telerehabilitation in surgical patients: a systematic review and meta-analysis. Physiotherapy. 2018;104(3):277–98. https://doi.org/10.1016/j.physio.2018.04.004.
10. Cottrell MA, Galea OA, O'Leary SP, Hill AJ, Russell TG. Real-time telerehabilitation for treating musculoskeletal conditions is effective and comparable to standard practice: a systematic review and meta-analysis. Clin Rehabil. 2016;31(5):625–38. https://doi.org/10.1177/0269215516645148.
11. Ceravolo MG, Arienti C, de Sire A, Andrenelli E, Negrini F, Lazzarini SG, et al. Rehabilitation and COVID-19: the cochrane rehabilitation 2020 rapid living systematic review. Eur J Phys Rehabil Med. 2020;56(5):642–51. https://doi.org/10.23736/s1973-9087.20.06501-6.
12. Halpin SJ, McIvor C, Whyatt G, Adams A, Harvey O, McLean L, et al. Postdischarge symptoms and rehabilitation needs in survivors of COVID-19 infection: a cross-sectional evaluation. J Med Virol. 2021;93(2):1013–22. https://doi.org/10.1002/jmv.26368.
13. Özden F, Arik AF, Tuğay N. Ortopedik Fizyoterapi Alanında Güncel Telerehabilitasyon Yaklaşımları. Turkiye Klinikleri J Health Sci. 2020;5(2):354–60.

14. Gilbert AW, Jaggi A, May CR. What is the patient acceptability of real-time 1:1 videoconferencing in an orthopaedics setting? A systematic review. Physiotherapy. 2018;104(2):178–86. https://doi.org/10.1016/j.physio.2017.11.217.
15. Rashedi E, Barati E. Telemedicine technologies and effectiveness: a review article. UMSHA-PSJ. 2013;11(3):1–8.
16. Yelin E, Weinstein S, King T. The burden of musculoskeletal diseases in the United States. Semin Arthritis Rheum. 2016;46(3):259–60. https://doi.org/10.1016/j.semarthrit.2016.07.013.
17. Lawford BJ, Delany C, Bennell KL, Hinman RS. "I was really sceptical…But it worked really well": a qualitative study of patient perceptions of telephone-delivered exercise therapy by physiotherapists for people with knee osteoarthritis. Osteoarthr Cartil. 2018;26(6):741–50. https://doi.org/10.1016/j.joca.2018.02.909.
18. Dario AB, Moreti Cabral A, Almeida L, Ferreira ML, Refshauge K, Simic M, et al. Effectiveness of telehealth-based interventions in the management of non-specific low back pain: a systematic review with meta-analysis. Spine J. 2017;17(9):1342–51. https://doi.org/10.1016/j.spinee.2017.04.008.
19. Jiang S, Xiang J, Gao X, Guo K, Liu B. The comparison of telerehabilitation and face-to-face rehabilitation after total knee arthroplasty: a systematic review and meta-analysis. J Telemed Telecare. 2016;24(4):257–62. https://doi.org/10.1177/1357633X16686748.
20. Werneke MW, Deutscher D, Grigsby D, Tucker CA, Mioduski JE, Hayes D. Telerehabilitation during the COVID-19 pandemic in outpatient rehabilitation settings: a descriptive study. Phys Ther. 2021;101(7):pzab110. https://doi.org/10.1093/ptj/pzab110.
21. Elgert L, Steiner B, Saalfeld B, Marschollek M, Wolf K-H. Health-enabling technologies to assist patients with musculoskeletal shoulder disorders when exercising at home: scoping review. JMIR Rehabil Assist Technol. 2021;8(1):e21107. https://doi.org/10.2196/21107.
22. Caffery LJ, Taylor M, North JB, Smith AC. Tele-orthopaedics: a snapshot of services in Australia. J Telemed Telecare. 2017;23(10):835–41. https://doi.org/10.1177/1357633X17732800.
23. Katz NB, Tenforde AS. Chapter 14—Telerehabilitation for musculoskeletal injuries. In: Alexander M, editor. Telerehabilitation. New Delhi: Elsevier; 2022. p. 197–212.
24. Chughtai M, Kelly JJ, Newman JM, Sultan AA, Khlopas A, Sodhi N, et al. The role of virtual rehabilitation in total and unicompartmental knee arthroplasty. J Knee Surg. 2019;32(01):105–10. https://doi.org/10.1055/s-0038-1637018.
25. Fiani B, Siddiqi I, Lee SC, Dhillon L. Telerehabilitation: development, application, and need for increased usage in the COVID-19 era for patients with spinal pathology. Cureus. 2020;12(9):e10563. https://doi.org/10.7759/cureus.10563.
26. Pramuka M, van Roosmalen L. Telerehabilitation technologies: accessibility and usability. Int J Telerehabil. 2009;1(1):85–98. https://doi.org/10.5195/ijt.2009.6016.
27. Borresen A, Wolfe C, Lin C-K, Tian Y, Raghuraman S, Nahrstedt K, et al. Usability of an immersive augmented reality based telerehabilitation system with haptics (ARTESH) for synchronous remote musculoskeletal examination. Int J Telerehabil. 2019;11(1):23–32. https://doi.org/10.5195/ijt.2019.6275.
28. Brewer BR, McDowell SK, Worthen-Chaudhari LC. Poststroke upper extremity rehabilitation: a review of robotic systems and clinical results. Top Stroke Rehabil. 2007;14(6):22–44. https://doi.org/10.1310/tsr1406-22.
29. Deutsch JE, Westcott MCS. Virtual reality and serious games in neurorehabilitation of children and adults: prevention, plasticity, and participation. Pediatr Phys Ther. 2017;29:S23–36.
30. Özden F, Özkeskin M, Tümtürk İ, Yalın Kılınç C. The effect of exercise and education combination via telerehabilitation in patients with chronic neck pain: a randomized controlled trial. Int J Med Inform. 2023;180:105281. https://doi.org/10.1016/j.ijmedinf.2023.105281.
31. Özden F, Güçlü B, Tümtürk İ, Doğrukök ÖN, İmerci A, Tuğay BU. The effect of visual feedback-based clinical monitoring application in patients with chronic low back pain: a randomized controlled trial. Eur Spine J. 2024; https://doi.org/10.1007/s00586-023-08098-1.

32. Tümtürk İ, Bakırhan S, Özden F, Gültaç E, Kılınç CY. The effect of telerehabilitation-based exercise and education on pain, function, strength, proprioception and psychosocial parameters in patients with knee osteoarthritis: a randomized controlled clinical trial. Am J Phys Med Rehabil. 2023; https://doi.org/10.1097/phm.0000000000002335.
33. Luptak M, Dailey N, Juretic M, Rupper R, Hill RD, Hicken BL, et al. The Care Coordination Home Telehealth (CCHT) rural demonstration project: a symptom-based approach for serving older veterans in remote geographical settings. Rural Remote Health. 2010;10(2):1375.
34. Young Lance B, Foster L, Silander A, Wakefield Bonnie J. Home telehealth: patient satisfaction, program functions, and challenges for the care coordinator. J Gerontol Nurs. 2011;37(11):38–46. https://doi.org/10.3928/00989134-20110706-02.
35. Amin J, Ahmad B, Amin S, Siddiqui AA, Alam MK. Rehabilitation professional and patient satisfaction with telerehabilitation of musculoskeletal disorders: a systematic review. Biomed Res Int. 2022;2022:7366063. https://doi.org/10.1155/2022/7366063.
36. Tenforde AS, Hefner JE, Kodish-Wachs JE, Iaccarino MA, Paganoni S. Telehealth in physical medicine and rehabilitation: a narrative review. PM R. 2017;9(5S):S51–S8. https://doi.org/10.1016/j.pmrj.2017.02.013.
37. Howard IM, Kaufman MS. Telehealth applications for outpatients with neuromuscular or musculoskeletal disorders. Muscle Nerve. 2018;58(4):475–85. https://doi.org/10.1002/mus.26115.
38. Turolla A, Rossettini G, Viceconti A, Palese A, Geri T. Musculoskeletal physical therapy during the COVID-19 pandemic: is telerehabilitation the answer? Phys Ther. 2020;100(8):1260–4. https://doi.org/10.1093/ptj/pzaa093.
39. Mehendale P, Iyenagar M, Bhatt G, Manwadkar S. Virtually administered intervention through telerehabilitation for chronic non-specific low Back pain: a review of literature. Cureus. 2023;15(8):e42942. https://doi.org/10.7759/cureus.42942.
40. Sarig Bahat H, Levy A, Yona T. The association between forward head posture and non-specific neck pain: a cross-sectional study. Physiother Theory Pract. 2023;39(8):1736–45. https://doi.org/10.1080/09593985.2022.2044420.
41. Derakhshanrad N, Yekaninejad MS, Mehrdad R, Saberi H. Neck pain associated with smartphone overuse: cross-sectional report of a cohort study among office workers. Eur Spine J. 2021;30(2):461–7. https://doi.org/10.1007/s00586-020-06640-z.
42. Özel M, Kaya Ciddi P. The effectiveness of telerehabilitation-based structured exercise therapy for chronic nonspecific neck pain: a randomized controlled trial. J Telemed Telecare. 2022; https://doi.org/10.1177/1357633X221095782.
43. Güngör F, Ovacık U, Ertan Harputlu Ö, Yekdaneh AA, Kurt İ, Ertürk Uzunoğlu G, et al. Tele-assessment of core performance and functional capacity: reliability, validity, and feasibility in healthy individuals. J Telemed Telecare. 2022; https://doi.org/10.1177/1357633X221117335.
44. Onan D, Ulger O, Martelletti P. Effects of spinal stabilization exercises delivered using telerehabilitation on outcomes in patients with chronic neck pain: a randomized controlled trial. Expert Rev Neurother. 2023;23(3):269–80. https://doi.org/10.1080/14737175.2023.2192870.
45. Özlü A, Ünver G, Tuna Hİ, Erdoğan A. Effects of interactive telerehabilitation practices in office workers with chronic nonspecific neck pain: randomized controlled study. Telemed eHealth. 2023; https://doi.org/10.1089/tmj.2023.0018.
46. Timurtaş E, Selçuk H, Uğur Canöz E, Inceer M, Batar S, Demirbüken İ, et al. Synchronous and asynchronous telerehabilitation methods produce similar benefits in individuals with non-specific neck pain. Arch Orthop Trauma Surg. 2024;144(2):559–66. https://doi.org/10.1007/s00402-023-05083-7.
47. Ye G, Koh RGL, Jaiswal K, Soomal H, Kumbhare D. The use of virtual reality in the rehabilitation of chronic nonspecific neck pain: a systematic review and meta-analysis. Clin J Pain. 2023;39(9):491–500.

48. Guo Q, Zhang L, Gui C, Chen G, Chen Y, Tan H, et al. Virtual reality intervention for patients with neck pain: systematic review and meta-analysis of randomized controlled trials. J Med Internet Res. 2023;25:e38256. https://doi.org/10.2196/38256.
49. Blanpied PR, Gross AR, Elliott JM, Devaney LL, Clewley D, Walton DM, et al. Neck pain: revision 2017. J Orthop Sports Phys Ther. 2017;47(7):A1–A83. https://doi.org/10.2519/jospt.2017.0302.
50. Patrick JO, Clint TM, Niamh LM, Simone JJMV, Scott DT, Helena B, et al. Which specific modes of exercise training are most effective for treating low back pain? Network meta-analysis. Br J Sports Med. 2020;54(21):1279. https://doi.org/10.1136/bjsports-2019-100886.
51. Sato T, Shimizu K, Shiko Y, Kawasaki Y, Orita S, Inage K, et al. Effects of Nintendo ring fit adventure exergame on pain and psychological factors in patients with chronic low Back pain. Games Health J. 2021;10(3):158–64. https://doi.org/10.1089/g4h.2020.0180.
52. Stamm O, Dahms R, Reithinger N, Ruß A, Müller-Werdan U. Virtual reality exergame for supplementing multimodal pain therapy in older adults with chronic back pain: a randomized controlled pilot study. Virtual Reality. 2022;26(4):1291–305. https://doi.org/10.1007/s10055-022-00629-3.
53. Meinke A, Peters R, Knols R, Karlen W, Swanenburg J. Exergaming using postural feedback from wearable sensors and exercise therapy to improve postural balance in people with nonspecific low back pain: protocol for a factorial pilot randomized controlled trial. JMIR Res Protoc. 2021;10(8):e26982. https://doi.org/10.2196/26982.
54. Collado-Mateo D, Merellano-Navarro E, Olivares PR, García-Rubio J, Gusi N. Effect of exergames on musculoskeletal pain: a systematic review and meta-analysis. Scand J Med Sci Sports. 2018;28(3):760–71. https://doi.org/10.1111/sms.12899.
55. Ditchburn J-L, van Schaik P, Dixon J, MacSween A, Martin D. The effects of exergaming on pain, postural control, technology acceptance and flow experience in older people with chronic musculoskeletal pain: a randomised controlled trial. BMC Sports Sci Med Rehabil. 2020;12(1):63. https://doi.org/10.1186/s13102-020-00211-x.
56. Mbada C, Olaoye M, Ayanniyi O, Johnson O, Odole A, Dada O. Comparative efficacy of clinic-based and telerehabilitation application of McKenzie therapy in low-back pain. Arch Phys Med Rehabil. 2017;98(10):e46–e7. https://doi.org/10.1016/j.apmr.2017.08.143.
57. Mbada CE, Olaoye MI, Dada OO, Ayanniyi O, Johnson OE, Odole AC, et al. Comparative efficacy of clinic-based and telerehabilitation application of McKenzie therapy in chronic low-back pain. Int J Telerehabil. 2019;11(1):41–58. https://doi.org/10.5195/ijt.2019.6260.
58. Fatoye F, Gebrye T, Fatoye C, Mbada CE, Olaoye MI, Odole AC, et al. The clinical and cost-effectiveness of telerehabilitation for people with nonspecific chronic low back pain: randomized controlled trial. JMIR Mhealth Uhealth. 2020;8(6):e15375. https://doi.org/10.2196/15375.
59. Villatoro-Luque FJ, Rodríguez-Almagro D, Aibar-Almazán A, Fernández-Carnero S, Pecos-Martín D, Ibáñez-Vera AJ, et al. Telerehabilitation for the treatment in chronic low back pain: a randomized controlled trial. J Telemed Telecare. 2023; https://doi.org/10.1177/1357633X231195091.
60. Villatoro-Luque FJ, Rodríguez-Almagro D, Aibar-Almazán A, Fernández-Carnero S, Pecos-Martín D, Ibáñez-Vera AJ, et al. In non-specific low back pain, is an exercise program carried out through telerehabilitation as effective as one carried out in a physiotherapy center? A controlled randomized trial. Musculoskelet Sci Pract. 2023;65:102765. https://doi.org/10.1016/j.msksp.2023.102765.
61. Okudan B, Çelik D, Koban O. The effectiveness of telerehabilitation-based exercise combined with pain neuroscience education for patients with facet joint arthrosis: a randomized controlled study. Eur J Pain. 2024;28(3):382–95. https://doi.org/10.1002/ejp.2187.
62. Starzec-Proserpio M, Vandyken C. Telerehabilitation for persistent pelvic girdle pain within a biopsychosocial framework—a case report. Physiother Theory Pract. 2023;39(10):2251–61. https://doi.org/10.1080/09593985.2022.2069618.
63. Özden F, Sarı Z, Karaman ÖN, Aydoğmuş H. The effect of video exercise-based telerehabilitation on clinical outcomes, expectation, satisfaction, and motivation in patients with chronic

low back pain. Irish J Med Sci (1971–). 2022;191(3):1229–39. https://doi.org/10.1007/s11845-021-02727-8.

64. Amorim P, Paulo JR, Silva PA, Peixoto P, Castelo-Branco M, Martins H. Machine learning applied to low back pain rehabilitation—a systematic review. Int J Digit Health. 2021;1(1):10.
65. Dobija L, Lechauve J-B, Mbony-Irankunda D, Plan-Paquet A, Dupeyron A, Coudeyre E. Smartphone applications are used for self-management, telerehabilitation, evaluation and data collection in low back pain healthcare: a scoping review. F1000Res. 2024;11:1001.
66. Hornung AL, Rudisill SS, Suleiman RW, Siyaji ZK, Sood S, Siddiqui S, et al. Low back pain: what is the role of YouTube content in patient education? J Orthop Res. 2022;40(4):901–8. https://doi.org/10.1002/jor.25104.
67. Moraes ÍA, Cardoso A, Soares AB, de Oliveira DAR, Júnior EL. Combining immersive virtual reality and postural therapy for scoliosis treatment and prevention in children. Res Biomed Eng. 2022;38(3):1003–16. https://doi.org/10.1007/s42600-022-00235-x.
68. Song Y. A brief review of the development of telerehabilitation and its application in patients of adolescent idiopathic scoliosis. Biomed J Sci Tech Res. 2023;48(2):39576–82.
69. Bottino L, Settino M, Promenzio L, Cannataro M. Scoliosis management through apps and software tools. Int J Environ Res Public Health. 2023; https://doi.org/10.3390/ijerph20085520.
70. Ahmad F, Wang MY. Spinal deformity? There's an app for that! World Neurosurg. 2013;80(5):446–7. https://doi.org/10.1016/j.wneu.2013.09.011.
71. Samad-Soltani T, Heshmati A, Hazrati H, Salahzade ZS, Hachesu PR, Ekrami NK. The effectiveness of mobile-learning in teaching corrective exercises to scoliosis patients: a quasi-experimental study. Res Square. 2021; https://doi.org/10.21203/rs.3.rs-931752/v1.
72. Cozeta Anca M, Mircea B, Radu VC. Scoliosis therapy, a study between the Schroth-3D method (held in the rehabilitation center) and Schroth-3D Teletherapy program. Sci Mov Health. 2021;21:361–70.
73. Manzak Dursun AS, Ozyilmaz S, Ucgun H, Elmadag NM. The effect of pilates-based exercise applied with hybrid telerehabilitation method in children with adolescent idiopathic scoliosis: a randomized clinical trial. Eur J Pediatr. 2023; https://doi.org/10.1007/s00431-023-05340-2.
74. Marin L, Albanese I, Gentile FL, Patanè P, Manzoni F, Pedrotti L, et al. Scoliosis: online exercises versus telerehabilitation. A feasibility trial. Minerva. 2021;72(3):313–21.
75. Park J-H, Stegall P, Roye D, Agrawal S. Robotic Spine Exoskeleton (RoSE): characterizing the three-dimensional stiffness of the human torso in the treatment of spine deformity. In: IEEE transactions on neural systems and rehabilitation engineering. 2018; p. 1. https://doi.org/10.1109/TNSRE.2018.2821652.
76. Steiner B, Elgert L, Saalfeld B, Schwartze J, Borrmann HP, Kobelt-Pönicke A, et al. Health-enabling technologies for telerehabilitation of the shoulder: a feasibility and user acceptance study. Methods Inf Med. 2020;59(S02):e90–9. https://doi.org/10.1055/s-0040-1713685.
77. Clark RA, Mentiplay BF, Hough E, Pua YH. Three-dimensional cameras and skeleton pose tracking for physical function assessment: a review of uses, validity, current developments and Kinect alternatives. Gait Posture. 2019;68:193–200. https://doi.org/10.1016/j.gaitpost.2018.11.029.
78. Ongvisatepaiboon K, Chan JH, Vanijja V. Smartphone-based tele-rehabilitation system for frozen shoulder using a machine learning approach. In: 2015 IEEE symposium series on computational intelligence; 2015. p. 811–5.
79. Tousignant M, Giguère AM, Morin M, Pelletier J, Sheehy A, Cabana F. In-home telerehabilitation for proximal humerus fractures: a pilot study. Int J Telerehabil. 2014;6(2):31–7. https://doi.org/10.5195/ijt.2014.6158.
80. Carbonaro N, Lucchesi I, Lorusssi F, Tognetti A. Tele-monitoring and tele-rehabilitation of the shoulder muscular-skeletal diseases through wearable systems. In: 2018 40th Annual international conference of the IEEE Engineering in Medicine and Biology Society (EMBC); 2018. p. 4410–3.
81. Palm KB, Blazar PE, Manna JC, Serig AS, Phillips EA, Bay CP, et al. Feasibility, effectiveness and patient satisfaction of telerehabilitation after thumb carpometacarpal arthroplasty

and reverse total shoulder arthroplasty: a pilot study. J Telemed Telecare. 2021;29(7):521–9. https://doi.org/10.1177/1357633X21999578.
82. Eriksson L, Lindström B, Ekenberg L. Patients' experiences of telerehabilitation at home after shoulder joint replacement. J Telemed Telecare. 2011;17(1):25–30. https://doi.org/10.1258/jtt.2010.100317.
83. Pastora-Bernal JM, Martín-Valero R, Barón-López FJ, Moyano NG, Estebanez-Pérez M-J. Telerehabilitation after arthroscopic subacromial decompression is effective and not inferior to standard practice: preliminary results. J Telemed Telecare. 2017;24(6):428–33. https://doi.org/10.1177/1357633X17706583.
84. Malliaras P, Cridland K, Hopmans R, Ashton S, Littlewood C, Page R, et al. Internet and telerehabilitation-delivered management of rotator cuff–related shoulder pain (INTEL Trial): randomized controlled pilot and feasibility trial. JMIR Mhealth Uhealth. 2020;8(11):e24311. https://doi.org/10.2196/24311.
85. Camargo PR, Policastro PO, Gava V. Chapter 16—Telerehabilitation in patients with frozen shoulder. In: Struyf F, editor. Frozen shoulder. Academic Press; 2024. p. 231–41.
86. Bansal S, Anand B, Gupta M, Solanki I. Effectiveness of exercises by telerehabilitation for neck and shoulder rehabilitation: a scoping review. PriMera Sci Surg Res Pract. 2023;1(1):3–9.
87. Gava V, Ribeiro LP, Barreto RPG, Camargo PR. Effectiveness of physical therapy given by telerehabilitation on pain and disability of individuals with shoulder pain: a systematic review. Clin Rehabil. 2022;36(6):715–25. https://doi.org/10.1177/02692155221083496.
88. Suero-Pineda A, Oliva-Pascual-Vaca Á, Durán MR-P, Sánchez-Laulhé PR, García-Frasquet MÁ, Blanquero J. Effectiveness of a telerehabilitation evidence-based tablet app for rehabilitation in traumatic bone and soft tissue injuries of the hand, wrist, and fingers. Arch Phys Med Rehabil. 2023;104(6):932–41. https://doi.org/10.1016/j.apmr.2023.01.016.
89. Staszuk A, Wiatrak B, Tadeusiewicz R, Karuga-Kuźniewska E, Rybak Z. Telerehabilitation approach for patients with hand impairment. Acta Bioeng Biomech. 2016;18(4):55–62.
90. Abedi A, Colella TJF, Pakosh M, Khan SS. Artificial intelligence-driven virtual rehabilitation for people living in the community: a scoping review. NPJ Digit Med. 2024;7(1):25. https://doi.org/10.1038/s41746-024-00998-w.
91. Placidi G. A smart virtual glove for the hand telerehabilitation. Comput Biol Med. 2007;37(8):1100–7. https://doi.org/10.1016/j.compbiomed.2006.09.011.
92. Cortese M, Cempini M, Ribeiro PRA, Soekadar SR, Carrozza MC, Vitiello N. A mechatronic system for robot-mediated hand telerehabilitation. IEEE/ASME Trans Mechatron. 2015;20(4):1753–64. https://doi.org/10.1109/TMECH.2014.2353298.
93. Airò Farulla G, Pianu D, Cempini M, Cortese M, Russo LO, Indaco M, et al. Vision-based pose estimation for robot-mediated hand telerehabilitation. Sensors. 2016; https://doi.org/10.3390/s16020208.
94. Placidi G, Di Matteo A, Lozzi D, Polsinelli M, Theodoridou E. Patient-therapist cooperative hand telerehabilitation through a novel framework involving the virtual glove system. Sensors. 2023; https://doi.org/10.3390/s23073463.
95. Giansanti D, Morelli S, Maccioni G, Lanzetta M, Macellari V. Health technology assessment of a homecare device for telemonitoring and telerehabilitation for patients after hand transplantation. Telemed eHealth. 2008;14(1):69–75. https://doi.org/10.1089/tmj.2007.0023.
96. Núñez-Cortés R, Cruz-Montecinos C, Torreblanca-Vargas S, Tapia C, Gutiérrez-Jiménez M, Torres-Gangas P, et al. Effectiveness of adding pain neuroscience education to telerehabilitation in patients with carpal tunnel syndrome: a randomized controlled trial. Musculoskelet Sci Pract. 2023;67:102835. https://doi.org/10.1016/j.msksp.2023.102835.
97. Suero-Pineda A, Oliva-Pascual-Vaca A, Rodríguez-Piñero Durán M, Rodríguez Sánchez-Laulhé P, García-Frasquet MA, Blanquero J. Effectiveness of a tablet telerehabilitation application in patients with distal radius fracture. Rehabilitacion (Madr). 2024;58(1):100818. https://doi.org/10.1016/j.rh.2023.100818.
98. Pech-Argüelles RC, Miranda-Ortiz YJ, Velázquez-Hernández HE, Domínguez-Cordero R, Ruiz-PachecoJuan C, Figueroa-García J, et al. Tele-rehabilitation program in patients with

distal radius fracture: a controlled clinical trial. Cir Cir. 2023; https://doi.org/10.24875/ciru.22000328.

99. Mayer N, Portnoy S, Palti R, Levanon Y. The efficacy of tele-rehabilitation program for improving upper limb function among adults following elbow fractures: a pilot study. Appl Sci. 2021;11(4):1708. https://doi.org/10.3390/app11041708.
100. Svingen J, Rosengren J, Turesson C, Arner M. A smartphone application to facilitate adherence to home-based exercise after flexor tendon repair: a randomised controlled trial. Clin Rehabil. 2020;35(2):266–75. https://doi.org/10.1177/0269215520962287.
101. Antón D, Nelson M, Russell T, Goñi A, Illarramendi A. Validation of a Kinect-based telerehabilitation system with total hip replacement patients. J Telemed Telecare. 2015;22(3):192–7. https://doi.org/10.1177/1357633X15590019.
102. Eichler S, Salzwedel A, Rabe S, Mueller S, Mayer F, Wochatz M, et al. The effectiveness of telerehabilitation as a supplement to rehabilitation in patients after total knee or hip replacement: randomized controlled trial. JMIR Rehabil Assist Technol. 2019;6(2):e14236. https://doi.org/10.2196/14236.
103. Nelson M, Bourke M, Crossley K, Russell T. Telerehabilitation is non-inferior to usual care following total hip replacement—a randomized controlled non-inferiority trial. Physiotherapy. 2020;107:19–27. https://doi.org/10.1016/j.physio.2019.06.006.
104. Nelson M, Russell T, Crossley K, Bourke M, McPhail S. Cost-effectiveness of telerehabilitation versus traditional care after total hip replacement: a trial-based economic evaluation. J Telemed Telecare. 2019;27(6):359–66. https://doi.org/10.1177/1357633X19869796.
105. Kuether J, Moore A, Kahan J, Martucci J, Messina T, Perreault R, et al. Telerehabilitation for total hip and knee arthroplasty patients: a pilot series with high patient satisfaction. HSS J. 2019;15(3):221–5. https://doi.org/10.1007/s11420-019-09715-w.
106. Wu W-y, Y-g Z, Zhang Y-Y, Peng B, Xu W-g. Clinical effectiveness of home-based telerehabilitation program for geriatric hip fracture following total hip replacement. Orthop Surg. 2023;15(2):423–31. https://doi.org/10.1111/os.13521.
107. Zhang Y-Y, Zhang Y-G, Li Z, Li S-H, Xu W-G. Effect of home-based telerehabilitation on the postoperative rehabilitation outcome of hip fracture in the aging population. Orthop Surg. 2022;14(8):1768–77. https://doi.org/10.1111/os.13293.
108. Tsuge T, Yamamoto N, Taito S, Miura T, Shiratsuchi D, Yorifuji T. Efficacy of telerehabilitation for patients after hip fracture surgery: a systematic review and meta-analysis. J Telemed Telecare. 2023; https://doi.org/10.1177/1357633X231181632.
109. Sadiq S, Ahmad A, Ahmed A, Khan I, Asim HM, Aziz A. Role of tele-rehabilitation in patients following total hip replacement: systematic review of clinical trials. J Pak Med Assoc. 2022;72(1):101–7. https://doi.org/10.47391/jpma.832.
110. Ferrara PE, Codazza S, Ferriero G, Ricciardi D, Foti C, Maccauro G, et al. The effectiveness of telerehabilitation after hip or knee arthroplasty: a narrative review. J Biol Regul Homeost Agents. 2020;34(5 Suppl. 1):75–9.
111. Wang X, Hunter DJ, Vesentini G, Pozzobon D, Ferreira ML. Technology-assisted rehabilitation following total knee or hip replacement for people with osteoarthritis: a systematic review and meta-analysis. BMC Musculoskelet Disord. 2019;20(1):506. https://doi.org/10.1186/s12891-019-2900-x.
112. Tedesco S, Torre OM, Belcastro M, Torchia P, Alfieri D, Khokhlova L, et al. Design of a multi-sensors wearable platform for remote monitoring of knee rehabilitation. IEEE Access. 2022;10:98309–28. https://doi.org/10.1109/ACCESS.2022.3204969.
113. Nuevo M, Rodríguez-Rodríguez D, Jauregui R, Fabrellas N, Zabalegui A, Conti M, et al. Telerehabilitation following fast-track total knee arthroplasty is effective and safe: a randomized controlled trial with the ReHub® platform. Disabil Rehabil. 2024;46:2629–39. https://doi.org/10.1080/09638288.2023.2228689.
114. Piqueras M, Marco E, Coll M, Escalada F, Ballester A, Cinca C, et al. Effectiveness of an interactive virtual telerehabilitation system in patients after total knee arthoplasty: a randomized controlled trial. J Rehabil Med. 2013;45(4):392–6. https://doi.org/10.2340/16501977-1119.

115. Naeemabadi M, Fazlali H, Najafi S, Dinesen B, Hansen J. Telerehabilitation for patients with knee osteoarthritis: a focused review of technologies and teleservices. JMIR Biomed Eng. 2020;5(1):e16991. https://doi.org/10.2196/16991.
116. Jamwal PK, Hussain S, Mir-Nasiri N, Ghayesh MH, Xie SQ. Tele-rehabilitation using in-house wearable ankle rehabilitation robot. Assist Technol. 2018;30(1):24–33. https://doi.org/10.1080/10400435.2016.1230153.
117. Karime A, Al-Osman H, Alja'am JM, Gueaieb W, Saddik AE. Tele-wobble: a telerehabilitation wobble board for lower extremity therapy. IEEE Trans Instrum Meas. 2012;61(7):1816–24. https://doi.org/10.1109/TIM.2012.2192338.
118. Mohammadi N, Hadian M-R, Olyaei G-R. Comparison of the effects of Wii and conventional training on functional abilities and neurocognitive function in basketball-players with functional ankle instability: matched randomized clinical trial. Clin Rehabil. 2021;35(10):1454–64. https://doi.org/10.1177/02692155211010249.
119. Howells BE, Clark RA, Ardern CL, Bryant AL, Feller JA, Whitehead TS, et al. The assessment of postural control and the influence of a secondary task in people with anterior cruciate ligament reconstructed knees using a Nintendo Wii Balance Board. Br J Sports Med. 2013;47(14):914–9. https://doi.org/10.1136/bjsports-2012-091525.
120. Blasco J, Igual-Camacho C, Blasco M, Antón-Antón V, Ortiz-Llueca L, Roig-Casasús S. The efficacy of virtual reality tools for total knee replacement rehabilitation: a systematic review. Physiother Theory Pract. 2021;37(6):682–92. https://doi.org/10.1080/09593985.2019.1641865.
121. Manz WJ, Goel R, Fakunle OP, Labib SA, Bariteau JT. Feasibility of rapid development and deployment of a telemedicine program in a foot and ankle orthopedic practice. Foot Ankle Int. 2020;42(3):320–8. https://doi.org/10.1177/1071100720963059.
122. Correia FD, Molinos M, Neves C, Janela D, Carvalho D, Luis S, et al. Digital rehabilitation for acute ankle sprains: prospective longitudinal cohort study. JMIR Rehabil Assist Technol. 2021;8(3):e31247. https://doi.org/10.2196/31247.
123. Çil ET, Serif T, Şaylı U, Subaşı F. The effectiveness of "Dijital Steps" web based telerehabilitation system for patient with hindfoot pain: a randomised controlled trial. Foot. 2023;56:102040. https://doi.org/10.1016/j.foot.2023.102040.
124. Phuphanich ME, Sinha KR, Truong M, Pham QG. Telemedicine for musculoskeletal rehabilitation and orthopedic postoperative rehabilitation. Phys Med Rehabil Clin. 2021;32(2):319–53. https://doi.org/10.1016/j.pmr.2020.12.004.
125. Perez J, Niburski K, Stoopler M, Ingelmo P. Telehealth and chronic pain management from rapid adaptation to long-term implementation in pain medicine: a narrative review. Pain Rep. 2021;6(1):e912. https://doi.org/10.1097/pr9.0000000000000912.
126. Cranen K, Groothuis-Oudshoorn CGM, Vollenbroek-Hutten MMR, Ijzerman MJ. Toward patient-centered telerehabilitation design: understanding chronic pain patients' preferences for web-based exercise telerehabilitation using a discrete choice experiment. J Med Internet Res. 2017;19(1):e26. https://doi.org/10.2196/jmir.5951.

Teleassessment Methods in Neurologic Rehabilitation

3

Özgü İnal Özün, Mehmet Özkeskin, and Zekiye İpek Katirci Kirmaci

3.1 Teleassessment

Communication and information technologies offer new possibilities for clinical assessment. Specifically, Internet-based systems may address issues of accessibility and cost as one potential solution for the evaluation and monitoring of those patients who have a chronic disease, live in remote areas, prefer home-based care, and/or experience a loss of their independence [1]. However, since the COVID-19 pandemic, this process and long-term assessments for neurorehabilitation programs have sometimes become difficult. Therefore, self-assessment and telerehabilitation became reasonable alternatives for practitioners and patients as they could offer insight into the progress and maintenance of an adapted activity level. Due to the pandemic of the coronavirus disease 2019 (COVID-19), many consultations had to be postponed or delivered through telemedicine, especially for conditions causing long-term disability [2]. Research studies on adults with neurologic conditions have an even greater need to implement procedures for minimizing contact and maintaining social distancing, as a majority of individuals with stroke, multiple sclerosis, and spinal cord injury have comorbidities or factors (e.g., cardiovascular disease, diabetes, older age) that increase the risk for infection [3].

Ö. İnal Özün
Department of Physiotherapy and Rehabilitation, Gülhane Faculty of Physiotherapy and Rehabilitation, University of Health Sciences, Ankara, Turkey
e-mail: ozgu.inal@sbu.edu.tr

M. Özkeskin (✉)
Department of Physiotherapy and Rehabilitation, Faculty of Health Sciences, Ege University, İzmir, Turkey
e-mail: mehmet.ozkeskin@ege.edu.tr

Z. İ. K. Kirmaci
Department of Physiotherapy and Rehabilitation, Faculty of Health Sciences, Gaziantep Islam Science and Technology University, Gaziantep, Turkey

F. Özden et al. (eds.), *Telerehabilitation*, TELe-Health,
https://doi.org/10.1007/978-3-031-69080-8_3

Additionally, due to limitations with activities of daily living, challenges with transportation, and reliance on caregivers, individuals with neurological impairments face more significant challenges associated with multiple study visits. To this end, teleassessments and telerehabilitation are emerging as essential solutions for re-establishing research during and beyond the current pandemic [4]. Before embarking on remote assessments, in addition to ensuring the participant's access to the Internet, specific ethical considerations must also be addressed [5]. Key factors include participant privacy, confidentiality, informed consent, equitable access, and potential risks of remotely capturing data. Before beginning teleassessments, a discussion of risks and strategies to minimize risks and potential problems should be considered and incorporated into the consent process. Possible solutions to reduce risk may include utilizing secure software, procuring participant contact information in case of emergency, and ensuring that the participant has adequate functional ability to perform the assessment. After informed consent, the study staff can interview the participant regarding medical history and physical activity and determine whether the participant can safely progress to the remote assessment [5, 6]. Teleassessments are an emerging and promising strategy to recruit participants and establish baseline levels of function before in-person neurorehabilitation research or clinical visits [6]. Teleassessment techniques can inform healthcare professionals about patients' clinical status and improvements and allow professionals to collect real-time data on patients' progress remotely. Various remote assessment systems have been developed for teleassessment. Videoconferencing is convenient and reliable for evaluating patients with neurological symptoms [7, 8]. In one study, healthcare professionals and participants reported high satisfaction levels with telerehabilitation interventions in poststroke patients [9]. Principally, teleassessment is an interactive and real-time experience for the medical examiners and the inspected patients [10, 11], allowing visual, auditory, verbal, and even body language dynamics to be achieved by teleassessment as in the case of face-to-face evaluation [10, 11]. Remote monitoring and remote assessment are more complex than in-person assessment due to perceived safety risks, limited space in home settings, or the necessity of caregiver presence [6, 12, 13]. Although the evidence for the validity of such remote assessments is increasing [2, 14, 15].

3.2 Assessment Parameters According to the International Classification of Functioning, Disability, and Health

A common term for telecommunication technologies in healthcare is "digital health." Digital health in rehabilitation refers to using information and communication technology for assessment, monitoring, and care delivery. Examples of this technology include wearable sensors, activity trackers, smartphone applications, and telehealth platforms [16]. The use of communication technology to deliver rehabilitation services, such as clinical evaluations, health monitoring, and therapies, is known as telerehabilitation [17].

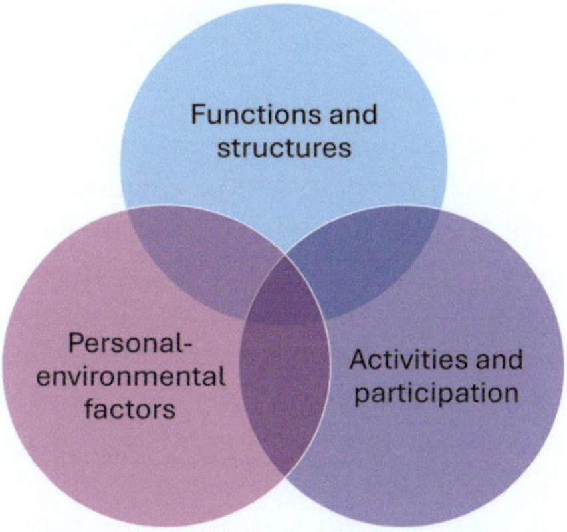

Fig. 3.1 Three main components of the ICF

Whether it comes to neurological illnesses, assessment and measurement play a critical role in choosing the best treatment program for physiotherapy and rehabilitation. In this sense, assessing people with neurological illnesses' physiological, physical, and social functioning might aid in the appropriate therapeutic decision-making process.

The International Classification of Functioning, Disability, and Health (ICF) is a classification that aims to create a shared, standard language and framework at the international level developed to describe health and health-related conditions. Using ICF in neurological physiotherapy and rehabilitation makes it possible to classify, more easily select, and interpret appropriate evaluation methods [14]. The three main components of the ICF emphasize how crucial it is for internal and external elements to interact and affect each person's health. These components are body functions and structures, activities and participation, and personal-environmental factors (Fig. 3.1). Body functions and structure impairments define issues with the structure and functioning of the body, such as a significant loss or deviation. Activity and participation limitation define difficulties a person might encounter when participating in life situations and carrying out daily tasks [15, 18, 19].

In this section, tele-evaluation methods that can be used in different neurological diseases will be presented within the framework of ICF.

3.3 Clinical Assessment Targeting Body Impairments

3.3.1 Motor

The absence of established remote assessment methods for neurological disorders impedes telerehabilitation in neurological settings by limiting clinicians' capacity to conduct objective and accurate clinical assessments remotely [20, 21]. Numerous remote evaluation studies have employed technology and robotic systems to review using synchronous and asynchronous applications, gaming, wide-angle cameras, desktop robot devices, sensors, mobile applications, and numerous technological platforms.

There are critical research gaps in neurological rehabilitation, explicitly addressing the feasibility and measuring features of remote lower extremity examinations. The main worry in remote gait and balance evaluation is that the participant's safety may be jeopardized (i.e., fall or injury) during functional testing, as well as the patient experiencing emotional distress owing to fear or frustration [6]. Wearable sensors and post-predictive algorithms based on video data enable administering tests such as the instrumented 6-Minute Walk Test and/or continuous remote monitoring of physical activity [22, 23]. However, such assessments are only viable in people who are well-functioning independent ambulators with a low risk of falling. As a result, participants should only be requested to complete activities that they are comfortable with and habitually perform at home on their own or with the assistance of a caregiver while utilizing assistive devices that they can use daily. It is recommended that evaluations be limited to tests that allow the subject to use their upper extremities for stability and where a support or sitting surface is easily accessible in case of a loss of balance [6].

In a study of individuals suffering from stroke [24], teleassessment of the Berg balance scale (BBS) and Motricity index (MI) measurement was found to be as effective as in-person evaluation. Nonetheless, the chair stand test (CST) proved insufficient for measurement. In the same way, it was discovered that tele-evaluation might replace face-to-face physical examinations in initial and follow-up evaluations of chronic patients. The Parkinson's DiaryR (daily activities, feelings, and general health status), Lift PulseR (tremor), PD MER (memory, balance, reaction time, and time perception), as well as the Movement Disorder Society Unified Parkinson Disease rating scale (MDS-UPDRS/CloudUPDRS APPs), are available on iOS and Android platforms [25]. Regarding PD teleassessment, several studies have shown that the motor component of the UPDRS may be completed reliably remotely [26]. However, the main worry is that people with Parkinson's disease are likely to be older, less adept at using technology, and have cognitive or physical disabilities that make interaction with the telemedicine platform more challenging. Remote evaluation has been proven less effective than face-to-face evaluation in evaluations involving the brainstem, cerebellar, and sensory functioning systems in Multiple Sclerosis (MS). Reflexes, gait, muscular tone and strength, and strength asymmetry are challenging to detect effectively during a virtual examination. Gait tests are often impossible unless the patient is assisted in situating the camera; patients with walking, balance, or coordination impairments risk falling [27]. A consensus has been reached on the differences in parts of the Expanded Disability Status Scale (EDSS) in multiple sclerosis between face-to-face and remote evaluations. However, a physical assessment requires assistance [28]. There have been few reports on telemedicine care for patients with neuromuscular illnesses. The ALS Functional Rating Scale-Revised (ALSFRSr) is commonly used to assess ALS progression. Some researchers have looked into the idea of an online self-administered version of the ALSFRSr scales, with good inter-rater reliability and low variability.

Beyond ALSFRSr, which may be readily assessed over the phone, remote neurological examination is also critical in treating ALS [29].

Many reviews revealed that in-person and remote examinations produced equivalent results, including improvements in upper extremity disability and function. There is a rising interest in developing remote assessments that can automatically and reliably monitor real-world functional usage of the afflicted arm. One of the most significant benefits of teleassessment is the ability to avoid interpreting the potential difference between objectively measured values in the clinic and how the patient perceives arm functionality [30, 31]. Research of stroke patients [32] found that the remote version of the upper extremity Fugl-Meyer evaluation is a promising instrument for examining upper extremity impairment in people with chronic stroke and moderate-to-severe arm impairment. A synchronized push-up teleassessment (e.g., videoconferencing, audio, or text-based interview) is a practical and valid method for determining maximum resistance strength in people with spinal cord injury (SCI) [33]. A study on Parkinson's patients [34] found that upper extremity teleassessment showed superior inter-subject reliability than face-to-face evaluation. The results reveal inter-rater solid reliability when comparing remote evaluation (function, agility, motor speed, tremor, and range of motion) to face-to-face assessment. A systematic review study examining remote evaluation of hand function in neurological disorders [34] found that it is possible to evaluate hand function in neurological disorders remotely. Telerehabilitation, particularly compatible with in-clinic measurements, and remote assessments via smartphone or tablet-based applications have been emphasized to ease the transition from clinic to home and speed up the remote diagnosis and treatment of hand function disorders.

In conclusion, the literature highlights the difficulties and inadequacy of studies on remote lower extremity assessments for neurorehabilitation research, critical gaps in the psychometric properties and clinical utility of the assessment tool used in the field of neurorehabilitation, and opportunities for future research to advance teleassessment. Furthermore, functional assessment is a challenge for telerehabilitation practice. The assessor should provide detailed instructions on the installation needed to ensure safety. The participant should be given standardized instructions outlining the space required for testing, the location of the camera for an unobstructed view, and how the activities should be carried out. A remote demo session on preparation, installation, and instructions may be necessary. Poor resolution of photos or recorded videos may impact data quality; thus, image settings must be improved during the practice/preparation session [6, 35, 36].

3.3.2 Non-Motor

Reports on examining sensory functions in neurological patients using a teleassessment method are minimal. In most research, sensory function has been employed as one of the subtests of a motor assessment tool. Neurological evaluation via audio-video connection has produced good results in reliability and validity in bedside examination, despite some limitations in assessing muscle tone, vibration sensitivity, and deep tendon reflexes [37, 38].

It has been demonstrated that remote examination yields lower evaluations of sensory functioning systems in MS patients than face-to-face examination. Visual acuity and direct vision of the optic nerve, eye movements (e.g., nystagmus), reflexes, and sensory asymmetry are all challenging to adequately detect during virtual testing [27]. Invisible MS symptoms, such as fatigue, cognitive impairment, or anxiety/depression, can be recognized by utilizing digital technology to create entirely new outcome measures gathered directly by patients in their everyday lives, hence increasing patient empowerment and involvement in clinical trials [39]. When using videoconferencing to collect updated information on a patient's health state and current functional level, a structured interview is advised to examine patients' self-reported MS symptoms (e.g., fatigue, pain, bowel/bladder symptoms). Patients should complete a symptom checklist (such as the Multiple Sclerosis Impact Scale) before their assessment. The possibility of remote EDSS evaluation in MS has been examined. However, an "in-home" technique comprising a vision card, tuning fork, pin, cotton swab, and alcohol swab is required with a caregiver to assist in the examination. It was established that several programs should be utilized to merge recordings from the "neuro kit" and wearable devices [40–42]. The American Academy of Neurology has suggested establishing a telemedicine service, indicating that general neurological examinations can be performed remotely, although with significant limitations. Comprehensive examinations of the eyes (e.g., fundoscopy), neuromuscular components (e.g., reflexes), and the vestibular system (e.g., Dix-Hallpike maneuver) are complex.

In contrast, evaluations of other neurological systems depend on the teleneurology setup and the availability of a caregiver to assist (e.g., sensory examination). Patient-reported outcome measures are entirely available online. Patient-determined disease steps (PDDS) were created as patient-reported outcome measures of disability in MS and have been validated for online use [43].

To gain insight into sensory systems, researchers taught caregivers how to use a needle or cotton swab to test for sensitivity and had them assessed via video assessment with adequate caregiver training for the remaining neurological symptoms (evaluation of balance and gait, performance of cerebellar tasks) thought to be crucial for these patients [44, 45]. They evaluated it this way [23, 24]. In another study, [46] proposed implementing the Veterans Affairs Neuropathy Scale (VANS), an excellent remote assessment instrument for diagnosing and monitoring the severity of polyneuropathies with appropriate sensitivity and specificity. However, it has been stated that this scale requires more confirmation beyond the pilot study. According to the polyneuropathy literature, the Veterans Affairs Neuropathy Scale can be successfully used via telemedicine to examine and monitor polyneuropathy symptoms in patients [46, 47]. This scale evaluates components such as gait, Romberg test, knee reflexes, and pinprick sensation, all partial components of a comprehensive spinal exam. However, in-person assistance is required to complete all portions of this examination correctly, limiting assessment completion to specific patient subgroups [48]. In certain circumstances, such as neuromuscular junction illness (e.g., Myasthenia Gravis), neurological evaluation requires repeating exercises that can be performed virtually to test for fatigue [49] and hence has certain limits.

3.3.3 Cognitive

The usage of telehealth techniques to measure cognitive functions has expanded dramatically. Given the widespread usage of technology in everyday contexts, cognitive assessment using information and communication technologies might be considered an ecologically valid technique for assessing human mental performance in specific situations. Evaluating cognitive function is critical so the participant can follow instructions throughout all evaluation instruments and processes, connect with the study team, and learn how to use videoconferencing technologies. Delivering cognitive evaluations remotely may make them more accessible to a larger audience [50].

Several studies indicate that people with cognitive disorders can be identified and monitored via video teleconferencing, video phones, and telephones. Regarding cerebral function, various neuropsychological tests have been studied for remote usage. However, there are few freely available standardized and verified remote cognitive screening techniques [50]. The Symbol Digit Modalities Test (SDMT) is strongly associated with disability progression and has been proposed as a screening test for cognitive impairment in MS [51]. The oral form of the SDMT has been certified for remote usage [52] and so can be efficiently utilized in tele-neurology. The Rowland Universal Dementia Assessment Scale (RUDAS) and Repeatable Battery for Neuropsychological Status (RBANS) have been validated for use with videoconferencing when compared to face-to-face assessment [53, 54]. Tests such as the Mini-Mental State Exam (MMSE) and the Montreal Cognitive Assessment (MOCA) have demonstrated higher accuracy in telehealth administration than in face-to-face administration [55, 56]. However, studies using cognitive tests have yielded varying results. Although MoCA, Telephone Interview for Cognitive Status, and the 26-point telephone version of the MMSE can be administered using telephones, these screening tools are not appropriate for early stroke-specific cognitive domains that are commonly affected. It has been highlighted that it was designed specifically for general dementia screening [57, 58]. Many of these tools require a paid license or educational qualification to access and use the materials.

Remote administration of cognitive testing presents challenges such as patients' sensorimotor limitations, distractions, room setup, connectivity issues, poor audio and video quality, volume control, camera setup, touch screen problems, and the individual's movement in front of the webcam. Some challenges may be alleviated by administering cognitive tests via video rather than telephone. However, most current studies in videoconferencing neuropsychological testing have focused on the feasibility of implementation. Although studies suggest that conducting some neuropsychological evaluations via videoconferencing [59] is feasible and acceptable, the correct interpretation of test scores is an important issue.

In addition to technology challenges, the noted drawback of Cognitive TeleAssessment across research is a loss of physical presence, which may result in a poorer understanding of nonverbal and implicit communication. These aspects reduce the operator-child contact and the need for re-engagement tactics (for example, imitation encouragement), which are frequently required in the evaluation of children, in particular [59]. However, information and communication technologies are regarded as feasible and reliable tools for implementing cognitive assessment because they can provide multi-sensory and motivating environments and increase compliance and participation, particularly in children, compared to traditional paper-and-pencil standardized tests [60]. However, remote assessment of children's cognitive development can only partially replace traditional in-person testing procedures. The child's age, attention level, engagement, adaptation, physical or sensory or mental impairments, personal history, environment, culture, ethnic group, and geographical region are all relevant considerations when selecting evaluation cognitive teleassessment instruments [61]. It is necessary to develop guidelines for the technological usage of cognitive teleassessment in children and improve personal requirements, evaluation criteria, and mental functions that can be assessed [53, 62].

Although older people are increasingly skilled at using technology, it is essential to consider age-related perceptual, linguistic, and cognitive limitations. Investigating how socioeconomic and economic issues influence the interpretation of distant cognitive assessments [63] is vital. Evaluation of telehealth requires clinician and patient comfort and technology proficiency, awareness of telehealth constraints, and a choice on when to move to a face-to-face encounter.

Despite results indicating that face-to-face neuropsychological testing is comparable to telemedicine, validation studies are still needed [63]. Furthermore, the efficacy of remote cognitive evaluations for diagnosis in real-world clinical practice and their measurement features in producing clinically relevant change over time is still being determined. Most instruments were designed for use in epidemiological research or clinical trials; therefore, they are best suited for quickly characterizing the cognitive functioning of a group rather than individual individuals. Most validation studies provide minimal information about test accuracy at the personal level, particularly in patients with complicated comorbidities or from different populations, because race/ethnicity has been proven to interact with the testing procedure. When deciding between telephone and videoconferencing testing, consider the patient's age and the Internet connection quality [64]. Confidentiality and data privacy are also essential considerations during cognitive teleassessment.

3.4 Clinical Assessment Targeting Activity and Participation Limitation

3.4.1 Activities of Daily Living

Even though telerehabilitation has recently become much more popular, rehabilitation specialists continue identifying obstacles to its adoption, including distance assessment.

When recording different motor impairments, such as balance, mobility, and upper extremity function, valid and reliable outcome measures are required in remote assessments. The psychometric qualities of musculoskeletal evaluations administered remotely, such as the Oswestry Disability Index and goniometry, have been documented in research [20, 21].

However, the need for validated remote assessment measures for neurological deficits makes it more difficult for clinicians to complete clinical assessments remotely objectively and accurately, hindering telerehabilitation implementation in neurological settings [65].

A review examining studies that performed tele-evaluation in neurological patients stated that although there were studies evaluating activity limitations, there were no studies assessing participation limitations with telerehabilitation. Studies are shown to evaluate functional mobility, walking and physical activity, upper extremity function including manipulation, grasping and releasing, and reaching, activities of daily living including balance, communication activities, and speech. Virtual reality technology, with or without wearable sensors or haptic systems, is the most commonly used system, followed by wearable sensors combined with or without mobile applications and synchronous telerehabilitation [66].

In the International Classification of Functioning, Disability, and Health (ICF), approved by the World Health Organization (WHO) in 2001, participation is defined as being in life, while participation limitations are defined as problems a person may encounter. Activities of Daily Living (ADL) are the tasks of eating and drinking, moving (transferring to a chair, bed, moving in bed, moving around the house, using stairs), going to the toilet, and performing personal hygiene tasks that people perform to protect their health and well-being and to live independently at home and in society. It includes activities such as (washing hair and body, oral hygiene, shaving), dressing, and undressing.

Participation in daily living activities is an important outcome measure of rehabilitation [67].

In ADL evaluations, in-bed activities, self-care activities, eating activities, dressing activities, wheelchair activities, walking and travel activities, and communication activities are evaluated.

In recent years, various telerehabilitation programs have been designed and studied to improve the abilities and independence of stroke patients living at home in daily living activities [68, 69].

With the development of today's technological age, teleassessment techniques enable professionals to collect real-time data about the development of patients remotely. Videoconferencing is a feasible and reliable method to evaluate patients with neurological symptoms [7].

Many standardized, valid, and reliable questionnaires have been developed to evaluate daily living activities. Questionnaires for neurological patients are as follows: Barthel Index, Functional Independence Scale, Modified Rankin Scale, Parkinson's Activity Scale, Activity-Specific Balance Confidence Scale, and Rivermead Mobility Index [70–75].

3.4.2 Activity Participation

ICF, aiming to create a shared, standard language and framework for describing health and health-related situations, has defined health domains and health-related areas in two lists: from the body and society/individual perspectives. Mainly covered are body functions and structures, activities, and participation. Activity and participation, which the ICF states as a component for functioning and disability, covers all areas that mean functionality from individual and social perspectives. In the classification, "participation" is defined as being in life, and "participation limitations" are defined as problems that a person may encounter in life situations. Activities and participation fields are expressed as a single list in nine sections, and these fields can be used to indicate events or participation, or both. These sections include learning and applying knowledge, general tasks and demands, communication, relocation, self-care, home life, interpersonal interactions and relationships, basic living spaces, community life, social life, and citizenship [14]. The physical, cognitive, and psychological effects resulting from stroke can lead to a wide range of activity limitations and participation restrictions, even in a long-term perspective [76]. In particular, some studies have noted that social participation is very low in the first 3 months of discharge, with significant increases in the following few months [77]. In a systematic review study conducted by Ezekiel and colleagues, 82 studies were examined, and age, stroke severity, comorbidity, depression, cognitive level, balance, hand and arm function, aphasia, fatigue, and pain were reported as factors associated with participation [78]. A randomized controlled study in Brazil investigating the effect of cane use on walking and social participation in individuals with stroke stated that if walking increases, the benefits can be transferred to involvement. It has also been noted that individuals may gain more free physical activity at home and in the community, reduced disability, increased social interactions, and increased ability to participate in work and leisure activities [79]. It has been observed in the literature that in studies conducted on stroke patients, social participation assessment data were collected by interview technique or by using a participation scale. In a systematic review study conducted by Tse et al., 36 different participation scales were discussed [80]. The most frequently used of these scales are the Stroke Impact Scale (SIS), London Handicap Scale (LHS), Assessment of Life Habits (LIFEH), Frenchay Acitivities Index and Activity Card Sort (ACS). It has been stated that the scales that most cover ICF's activity and participation areas are LIFE-H, ACS, and SIS. Other scales are the Reintegration to Normal Living Index, the Impact on Participation and Autonomy Questionnaire, The Stroke-Specific Quality of Life Scale, and the World Health Organization Disability Assessment Chart 2.0 [81–89].

Due to functional and cognitive limitations, many activities of daily living (ADLs), such as dressing and eating, may be affected in individuals with neurological diseases [90]. In the neurological patient group who has long-term participation problems due to disorders, ADLs participation is among the treatment goals [91].

Rehabilitation aims to improve the quality of life by increasing the existing capacity of the individual. With the planned treatment programs, the symptoms are improved, and the individual aims to perform daily activities and participate in social life. It is possible to evaluate participation limitations and different areas of quality of life with quality-of-life surveys. Other questionnaires used in neurological diseases are: Canadian Occupational Performance Measurement, Short Form 36 Scale, Nottingham Health Profile, Parkinson's Disease Questionnaire, Multiple Sclerosis Quality of Life 54 Questionnaire, Individualized Neuromuscular Quality of Life Questionnaire, ALS-Specific Quality of Life [92–98].

Although individuals with neurological diseases are evaluated remotely with the specified scales in telerehabilitation interventions, it should be assessed whether there is a difference between the face-to-face application of these scales and whether the remote evaluation is valid and reliable.

References

1. Bernard M-M, Janson F, Flora PK, Faulkner GE, Meunier-Norman L, Fruhwirth M. Videoconference-based physiotherapy and tele-assessment for homebound older adults: a pilot study. Act Adapt Aging. 2009;33(1):39–48.
2. Moccia M, Lanzillo R, Brescia Morra V, Bonavita S, Tedeschi G, Leocani L, et al. Assessing disability and relapses in multiple sclerosis on tele-neurology. Neurol Sci. 2020;41:1369–71.
3. Yang J, Zheng Y, Gou X, Pu K, Chen Z, Guo Q, et al. Prevalence of comorbidities and its effects in patients infected with SARS-CoV-2: a systematic review and meta-analysis. Int J Infect Dis. 2020;94:91–5.
4. Richmond T, Peterson C, Cason J, Billings M, Terrell EA, Lee ACW, et al. American Telemedicine Association's principles for delivering telerehabilitation services. Int J Telerehabil. 2017;9(2):63.
5. Demiris G, Oliver DP, Courtney KL. Ethical considerations for the utilization of telehealth technologies in home and hospice care by the nursing profession. Nurs Adm Q. 2006;30(1):56–66.
6. Madhavan S, Sivaramakrishnan A, Bowden MG, Chumbler NR, Field-Fote EC, Kesar TM. Commentary: remote assessments of gait and balance-implications for research during and beyond COVID-19. Top Stroke Rehabil. 2022;29(1):74–81.
7. Craig J, Patterson V, Russell C, Wootton R. Interactive videoconsultation is a feasible method for neurological in-patient assessment. Eur J Neurol. 2000;7(6):699–702.
8. Handschu R, Littmann R, Reulbach U, Gaul C, Heckmann JG, Neundörfer B, et al. Telemedicine in emergency evaluation of acute stroke: interrater agreement in remote video examination with a novel multimedia system. Stroke. 2003;34(12):2842–6.
9. Johansson T, Wild C. Telerehabilitation in stroke care–a systematic review. J Telemed Telecare. 2011;17(1):1–6.
10. O'Cathail M, Sivanandan MA, Diver C, Patel P, Christian J. The use of patient-facing teleconsultations in the national health service: scoping review. JMIR Med Inform. 2020;8(3):e15380.
11. Winters JM. Telerehabilitation research: emerging opportunities. Annu Rev Biomed Eng. 2002;4(1):287–320.
12. Jansen-Kosterink S, Dekker-van Weering M, van Velsen L. Patient acceptance of a telemedicine service for rehabilitation care: a focus group study. Int J Med Inform. 2019;125:22–9.
13. Wentink M, van Bodegom-Vos L, Brouns B, Arwert H, Houdijk S, Kewalbansing P, et al. How to improve eRehabilitation programs in stroke care? A focus group study to identify requirements of end-users. BMC Med Inform Decis Mak. 2019;19:1–11.
14. World Health Organazation. https://www.who.int/standards/classifications/international-classification-of-functioning-disability-and-health. Accessed 10 Jan 2024.
15. International Classification of Functioning Disability and Health (ICF). https://www.physio-pedia.com/International_Classification_of_Functioning_Disability_and_Health_(ICF). Accessed 20 Jan 2024.

16. WHO. Recommendations on digital interventions for health system strengthening. WHO; 2019.
17. Parmanto B, Saptono A. Telerehabilitation: state-of-the-art from an informatics perspective. Int J Telerehabil. 2009;1(1):73.
18. A practical manual for using the international classification of functioning, disability and health. https://resources.relabhs.org/resource/a-practical-manual-for-using-the-international-classification-of-functioning-disability-and-health/. Accessed 20 Jan 2024.
19. International Classification of Functioning, Disability and Health (ICF). Beginners' guide. https://resources.relabhs.org/resource/international-classification-of-functioning-disability-and-health-icf-beginners-guide/. Accessed 20 Jan 2024.
20. Mani S, Sharma S, Omar B, Paungmali A, Joseph L. Validity and reliability of Internet-based physiotherapy assessment for musculoskeletal disorders: a systematic review. J Telemed Telecare. 2017;23(3):379–91.
21. Peyrusqué E, Granet J, Pageaux B, Buckinx F, Aubertin-Leheudre M. Assessing physical performance in older adults during isolation or lockdown periods: web-based video conferencing as a solution. J Nutr Health Aging. 2022;26:52–6.
22. Brooks GC, Vittinghoff E, Iyer S, Tandon D, Kuhar P, Madsen KA, et al. Accuracy and usability of a self-administered 6-minute walk test smartphone application. Circ Heart Fail. 2015;8(5):905–13.
23. Costa PHV, de Jesus TPD, Winstein C, Torriani-Pasin C, Polese JC. An investigation into the validity and reliability of mHealth devices for counting steps in chronic stroke survivors. Clin Rehabil. 2020;34(3):394–403.
24. Saral İ, SURUCU S, Yayla YT, Çakar E. Face-to-face assessment versus tele-assessment of chronic stroke patients: do the results meet the needs? J Health Sci Med. 2023;6(1):82–6.
25. Miele G, Straccia G, Moccia M, Leocani L, Tedeschi G, Bonavita S, et al. Telemedicine in Parkinson's disease: how to ensure patient needs and continuity of care at the time of COVID-19 pandemic. Telemed eHealth. 2020;26(12):1533–6.
26. Cubo E, Trejo Gabriel-Galán JM, Seco Martínez J, Rioja Alcubilla C, Yang C, Fernández Arconada O, et al. Comparison of office-based versus home web-based clinical assessments for Parkinson's disease. Mov Disord. 2012;27(2):308–11.
27. Giacomini PS, Oh J, Morrow SA, Beauchemin P, Clift F, Devonshire V. Videoconferencing and multiple sclerosis management: stopgap or stay tuned? Can J Neurol Sci. 2022;49(3):402–5.
28. Kane RL, Bever CT, Ehrmantraut M, Forte A, Culpepper WJ, Wallin MT. Teleneurology in patients with multiple sclerosis: EDSS ratings derived remotely and from hands-on examination. J Telemed Telecare. 2008;14(4):190–4.
29. Bakker LA, Schröder CD, Tan HH, Vugts SM, van Eijk RP, van Es MA, et al. Development and assessment of the inter-rater and intra-rater reproducibility of a self-administration version of the ALSFRS-R. J Neurol Neurosurg Psychiatry. 2020;91(1):75–81.
30. Essers B, Meyer S, De Bruyn N, Van Gils A, Boccuni L, Tedesco Triccas L, et al. Mismatch between observed and perceived upper limb function: an eye-catching phenomenon after stroke. Disabil Rehabil. 2019;41(13):1545–51.
31. Essers B, Coremans M, Veerbeek J, Luft A, Verheyden G. Daily life upper limb activity for patients with match and mismatch between observed function and perceived activity in the chronic phase post stroke. Sensors. 2021;21(17):5917.
32. Carmona C, Sullivan JE, Arceo R, Drogos J, Besser S, Gutierrez S, et al. Development and preliminary validity study of a modified version of the upper extremity Fugl-Meyer assessment for use in telerehabilitation. J Neurol Phys Ther. 2023;47(4):208–16.
33. Gomes Costa RR, Dorneles JR, Veloso JHCL, Gonçalves CWP, Neto FR. Feasibility and validity of the push-up test for synchronous and asynchronous strength tele-assessment in spinal cord injury individuals with paraplegia. J Spinal Cord Med. 2024;47:530–9.
34. Gopal A, Hsu W-Y, Allen DD, Bove R. Remote assessments of hand function in neurological disorders: systematic review. JMIR Rehabil Assist Technol. 2022;9(1):e33157.
35. Brito SAF, Scianni AA, Peniche PC, Faria CDCM. Measurement properties of outcome measures used in neurological telerehabilitation: a systematic review protocol. PLoS One. 2022;17(3):e0265841.

36. Chirra M, Marsili L, Wattley L, Sokol LL, Keeling E, Maule S, et al. Telemedicine in neurological disorders: opportunities and challenges. Telemed eHealth. 2019;25(7):541–50.
37. Pulley MT, Brittain R, Hodges W, Frazier C, Miller L, Matyjasik-Liggett M, et al. Multidisciplinary amyotrophic lateral sclerosis telemedicine care: the store and forward method. Muscle Nerve. 2019;59(1):34–9.
38. Awadallah M, Janssen F, Körber B, Breuer L, Scibor M, Handschu R. Telemedicine in general neurology: interrater reliability of clinical neurological examination via audio-visual telemedicine. Eur Neurol. 2019;80(5–6):289–94.
39. De Angelis M, Lavorgna L, Carotenuto A, Petruzzo M, Lanzillo R, Brescia Morra V, et al. Digital technology in clinical trials for multiple sclerosis: systematic review. J Clin Med. 2021;10(11):2328.
40. Lavorgna L, Brigo F, Moccia M, Leocani L, Lanzillo R, Clerico M, et al. e-Health and multiple sclerosis: an update. Mult Scler J. 2018;24(13):1657–64.
41. Yeroushalmi S, Maloni H, Costello K, Wallin MT. Telemedicine and multiple sclerosis: a comprehensive literature review. J Telemed Telecare. 2020;26(7–8):400–13.
42. Bove R, Bevan C, Crabtree E, Zhao C, Gomez R, Garcha P, et al. Toward a low-cost, in-home, telemedicine-enabled assessment of disability in multiple sclerosis. Mult Scler J. 2019;25(11):1526–34.
43. Lavorgna L, Sparaco M, Esposito S, Motl RW, Gallo A, Bisecco A, et al. Validity and reproducibility of the Italian version of the patient determined disease steps scale in people with multiple sclerosis. Mult Scler Relat Disord. 2017;18:173–6.
44. Kleyweg RP, Van Der Meché FG, Schmitz PI. Interobserver agreement in the assessment of muscle strength and functional abilities in Guillain-Barré syndrome. Muscle Nerve. 1991;14(11):1103–9.
45. Saporta MA, Granit V, Lewis R, Benatar M. Yes, we can: neuromuscular examination by telemedicine. Muscle Nerve. 2020;62(6):E83–E5.
46. Wilson AM, Ong MK, Saliba D, Jamal NI. The veterans affairs neuropathy scale: a reliable, remote polyneuropathy exam. Front Neurol. 2019;10:1050.
47. Wilson AM, Jamal NI, Cheng EM, Inkelas M, Saliba D, Hanssen A, et al. Teleneurology clinics for polyneuropathy: a pilot study. J Neurol. 2020;267:479–90.
48. Piche J, Butt BB, Ahmady A, Patel R, Aleem I. Physical examination of the spine using telemedicine: a systematic review. Global Spine J. 2021;11(7):1142–7.
49. Spina E, Trojsi F, Tozza S, Iovino A, Iodice R, Passaniti C, et al. How to manage with telemedicine people with neuromuscular diseases? Neurol Sci. 2021;42(9):3553–9.
50. Webb SS, Kontou E, Demeyere N. The COVID-19 pandemic altered the modality, but not the frequency, of formal cognitive assessment. Disabil Rehabil. 2022;44(21):6365–73.
51. Wojcik CM, Beier M, Costello K, DeLuca J, Feinstein A, Goverover Y, et al. Computerized neuropsychological assessment devices in multiple sclerosis: a systematic review. Mult Scler J. 2019;25(14):1848–69.
52. Silva P, Spedo C, Barreira AA, Leoni RF. Symbol digit modalities test adaptation for magnetic resonance imaging environment: a systematic review and meta-analysis. Mult Scler Relat Disord. 2018;20:136–43.
53. Galusha-Glasscock JM, Horton DK, Weiner MF, Cullum CM. Video teleconference administration of the repeatable battery for the assessment of neuropsychological status. Arch Clin Neuropsychol. 2016;31(1):8–11.
54. Wong L, Martin-Khan M, Rowland J, Varghese P, Gray LC. The Rowland Universal Dementia Assessment Scale (RUDAS) as a reliable screening tool for dementia when administered via videoconferencing in elderly post-acute hospital patients. J Telemed Telecare. 2012;18(3):176–9.
55. McEachern W, Kirk A, Morgan DG, Crossley M, Henry C. Reliability of the MMSE administered in-person and by telehealth. Can J Neurol Sci. 2008;35(5):643–6.
56. Wong A, Nyenhuis D, Black SE, Law LS, Lo ES, Kwan PW, et al. Montreal Cognitive Assessment 5-minute protocol is a brief, valid, reliable, and feasible cognitive screen for telephone administration. Stroke. 2015;46(4):1059–64.

57. Brandt J, Spencer M, Folstein M. The telephone interview for cognitive status. Neuropsychiatry Neuropsychol Behav Neurol. 1988;1(2):111–7.
58. Newkirk LA, Kim JM, Thompson JM, Tinklenberg JR, Yesavage JA, Taylor JL. Validation of a 26-point telephone version of the Mini-Mental State Examination. J Geriatr Psychiatry Neurol. 2004;17(2):81–7.
59. Raman N, Nagarajan R, Venkatesh L, Monica DS, Ramkumar V, Krumm M. School-based language screening among primary school children using telepractice: a feasibility study from India. Int J Speech Lang Pathol. 2019;21(4):425–34.
60. Luciana M, Nelson CA. Assessment of neuropsychological function through use of the Cambridge Neuropsychological Testing Automated Battery: performance in 4-to 12-year-old children. Dev Neuropsychol. 2002;22(3):595–624.
61. Ruffini C, Tarchi C, Morini M, Giuliano G, Pecini C. Tele-assessment of cognitive functions in children: a systematic review. Child Neuropsychol. 2022;28(6):709–45.
62. Wadsworth HE, Dhima K, Womack KB, Hart J Jr, Weiner MF, Hynan LS, et al. Validity of teleneuropsychological assessment in older patients with cognitive disorders. Arch Clin Neuropsychol. 2018;33(8):1040–5.
63. Castanho TC, Amorim L, Zihl J, Palha JA, Sousa N, Santos NC. Telephone-based screening tools for mild cognitive impairment and dementia in aging studies: a review of validated instruments. Front Aging Neurosci. 2014;6:16.
64. Brearly TW, Shura RD, Martindale SL, Lazowski RA, Luxton DD, Shenal BV, et al. Neuropsychological test administration by videoconference: a systematic review and meta-analysis. Neuropsychol Rev. 2017;27:174–86.
65. Block VA, Pitsch E, Tahir P, Cree BA, Allen DD, Gelfand JM. Remote physical activity monitoring in neurological disease: a systematic review. PLoS One. 2016;11(4):e0154335.
66. O'Neil J, Barnes K, Morgan Donnelly E, Sheehy L, Sveistrup H. Identification and description of telerehabilitation assessments for individuals with neurological conditions: a scoping review. Digit Health. 2023;9:20552076231183233.
67. Legg LA, Lewis SR, Schofield-Robinson OJ, Drummond A, Langhorne P. Occupational therapy for adults with problems in activities of daily living after stroke. Cochrane Database Syst Rev. 2017;7:CD003585.
68. Brennan DM, Mawson S, Brownsell S. Telerehabilitation: enabling the remote delivery of healthcare, rehabilitation, and self management. Advanced technologies in rehabilitation. Stud Health Technol Inform. 2009;145:231–48.
69. Lai JC, Woo J, Hui E, Chan W. Telerehabilitation—a new model for community-based stroke rehabilitation. J Telemed Telecare. 2004;10(4):199–205.
70. Shah S, Vanclay F, Cooper B. Improving the sensitivity of the Barthel Index for stroke rehabilitation. J Clin Epidemiol. 1989;42(8):703–9.
71. Hamilton BB, Laughlin JA, Fiedler RC, Granger CV. Interrater reliability of the 7-level functional independence measure (FIM). Scand J Rehabil Med. 1994;26(3):115–9.
72. Quinn TJ, Dawson J, Walters MR, Lees KR. Reliability of the modified Rankin Scale: a systematic review. Stroke. 2009;40(10):3393–5.
73. Keus S, Nieuwboer A, Bloem B, Borm G, Munneke M. Clinimetric analyses of the modified Parkinson activity scale. Parkinsonism Relat Disord. 2009;15(4):263–9.
74. Powell LE, Myers AM. The activities-specific balance confidence (ABC) scale. J Gerontol Ser A Biol Med Sci. 1995;50(1):M28–34.
75. Hsieh C, Hsueh I, Mao H. Validity and responsiveness of the rivermead mobility index in stroke patients. Scand J Rehabil Med. 2000;32(3):140–2.
76. Törnbom K, Hadartz K, Sunnerhagen KS. Self-perceived participation and autonomy at 1-year post stroke: a part of the stroke arm longitudinal study at the University of Gothenburg (SALGOT Study). J Stroke Cerebrovasc Dis. 2018;27(4):1115–22.
77. Kossi O, Nindorera F, Adoukonou T, Penta M, Thonnard J-L. Determinants of social participation at 1, 3, and 6 months poststroke in Benin. Arch Phys Med Rehabil. 2019;100(11):2071–8.

78. Ezekiel L, Collett J, Mayo NE, Pang L, Field L, Dawes H. Factors associated with participation in life situations for adults with stroke: a systematic review. Arch Phys Med Rehabil. 2019;100(5):945–55.
79. Avelino PR, Nascimento LR, Menezes KK, Scianni AA, Ada L, Teixeira-Salmela LF. Effect of the provision of a cane on walking and social participation in individuals with stroke: protocol for a randomized trial. Braz J Phys Ther. 2018;22(2):168–73.
80. Tse T, Douglas J, Lentin P, Carey L. Measuring participation after stroke: a review of frequently used tools. Arch Phys Med Rehabil. 2013;94(1):177–92.
81. Duncan PW, Wallace D, Lai SM, Johnson D, Embretson S, Laster LJ. The stroke impact scale version 2.0: evaluation of reliability, validity, and sensitivity to change. Stroke. 1999;30(10):2131–40.
82. Jenkinson C, Mant J, Carter J, Wade D, Winner S. The London handicap scale: a re-evaluation of its validity using standard scoring and simple summation. J Neurol Neurosurg Psychiatry. 2000;68(3):365.
83. Roy-Bouthot K, Filiatrault P, Caron C, Gagnon M, Prémont S, Levasseur M. Modification of the assessment of life habits (LIFE-H m) to consider personalized satisfaction with participation in activities and roles: results from a construct validity study with older adults. Disabil Rehabil. 2014;36(9):737–43.
84. Schuling J, De Haan R, Limburg M, Groenier K. The Frenchay Activities Index. Assessment of functional status in stroke patients. Stroke. 1993;24(8):1173–7.
85. Katz N, Karpin H, Lak A, Furman T, Hartman-Maeir A. Participation in occupational performance: reliability and validity of the Activity Card Sort. OTJR Occup Particip Health. 2003;23(1):10–7.
86. Wood-Dauphinee S, Opzoomer M, Williams JI, Marchand B, Spitzer WO. Assessment of global function: the Reintegration to Normal Living Index. Arch Phys Med Rehabil. 1988;69(8):583–90.
87. Cardol M, de Jong B. Impact op participatie en autonomie (IPA). Handleiding en vragenlijst. Amsterdam: Afdeling Revalidatie, Academisch Medisch Centrum; 2001.
88. Post MW, Boosman H, Van Zandvoort MM, Passier PE, Rinkel GJ, Visser-Meily JM. Development and validation of a short version of the Stroke Specific Quality of Life Scale. J Neurol Neurosurg Psychiatry. 2011;82(3):283–6.
89. Federici S, Bracalenti M, Meloni F, Luciano JV. World Health Organization disability assessment schedule 2.0: an international systematic review. Disabil Rehabil. 2017;39(23):2347–80.
90. Gokalp H, Clarke M. Monitoring activities of daily living of the elderly and the potential for its use in telecare and telehealth: a review. Telemed eHealth. 2013;19(12):910–23.
91. World Health Organization. Neurological disorders: public health challenges. World Health Organization; 2006.
92. Carswell A, McColl MA, Baptiste S, Law M, Polatajko H, Pollock N. The Canadian Occupational Performance Measure: a research and clinical literature review. Can J Occup Ther. 2004;71(4):210–22.
93. Wiklund I. The Nottingham Health Profile—a measure of health-related quality of life. Scand J Prim Health Care Suppl. 1990;1:15–8.
94. Anderson C, Laubscher S, Burns R. Validation of the Short Form 36 (SF-36) health survey questionnaire among stroke patients. Stroke. 1996;27(10):1812–6.
95. Heiskanen S, Meriläinen P, Pietilä AM. Health-related quality of life–testing the reliability of the MSQOL-54 instrument among MS patients. Scand J Caring Sci. 2007;21(2):199–206.
96. Jenkinson C, Fitzpatrick R, Peto V, Greenhall R, Hyman N. The Parkinson's Disease Questionnaire (PDQ-39): development and validation of a Parkinson's disease summary index score. Age Ageing. 1997;26(5):353–7.
97. Vincent K, Carr A, Walburn J, Scott D, Rose M. Construction and validation of a quality of life questionnaire for neuromuscular disease (INQoL). Neurology. 2007;68(13):1051–7.
98. Bromberg MB. Quality of life in amyotrophic lateral sclerosis. Phys Med Rehabil Clin N Am. 2008;19(3):591–605.

Telerehabilitation Methods in Neurologic Rehabilitation

4

Mehmet Özkeskin, Ece Ekici, and Hakan Polat

4.1 Telerehabilitation Mechanisms in Neurologic Rehabilitation

The effectiveness of telerehabilitation has been demonstrated through numerous studies in individuals with neurological disorders [1–3]. Several theories are discussed in the literature [4] regarding the mechanism of forming these results. The effect mechanism of telerehabilitation in neurological disorders is based on principles of neuroplasticity and motor learning [5, 6]. Additionally, its increased accessibility compared to clinical settings and the enhancement of patient compliance through enjoyable, game-based applications contribute to the effect mechanism. Essentially, the effectiveness of an intervention is directly linked to the application frequency. Telerehabilitation presents a new perspective in overcoming challenges commonly encountered in neurorehabilitation, such as the inability to administer high-dose treatment, low patient compliance with therapy, and disadvantages associated with treatment provided in a clinical setting.

M. Özkeskin (✉)
Department of Physiotherapy and Rehabilitation, Faculty of Health Sciences, Ege University, İzmir, Turkey
e-mail: mehmet.ozkeskin@ege.edu.tr

E. Ekici
Department of Physiotherapy and Rehabilitation, Faculty of Health Sciences, Toros University, Mersin, Turkey

H. Polat
Department of Physiotherapy and Rehabilitation, Faculty of Health Sciences, Sanko University, Gaziantep, Turkey

F. Özden et al. (eds.), *Telerehabilitation*, TELe-Health,
https://doi.org/10.1007/978-3-031-69080-8_4

4.2 Different Methods in Telerehabilitation

Telehealth is a wide range of health technologies providing substantial clinical support for patients, relatives, and healthcare professionals. Telerehabilitation is a part of telehealth that offers various methods for patients, including telemonitoring, teleconference, or telementoring [7]. Technological developments have enhanced telerehabilitation interventions, particularly in the last 20 years. The most significant advantages of using telerehabilitation include solving distance and time problems, reducing financial difficulties resulting from transportation expenses, minimizing the average length of hospital stay, enhancing the quality of life due to increased satisfaction and comfort area, reducing the risk of transmission of viruses and infections during pandemics, such as COVID-19, and ensuring isolation [8]. Nowadays, telerehabilitation is considered a separate specialization and application area for physiotherapists. Physiotherapists who work in this field should have adequate knowledge of technology. After closely following technological innovations and current studies and having a good command of different methods, these professionals can prefer and use this method appropriately. Telerehabilitation is practiced in three different methods. These methods are image-based, sensor-based, and virtual technology-based.

Image-based telerehabilitation is the oldest method among the telerehabilitation methods. Moreover, it is mainly performed with the videoconferencing platform system. The level of evidence is high since it is the oldest and the most preferred method. Physiotherapists conveniently prefer it due to modules such as remote diagnosis, evaluation, training, and follow-up for the patient [9].

Sensor-based telerehabilitation is used less with telerehabilitation compared to the use of image-based telerehabilitation together with telerehabilitation. In sensor-based telerehabilitation, the patient's movements are recorded through inertial sensors, including accelerometers and gyroscopes [10].

Virtual reality-based telerehabilitation systems are also called game-based telerehabilitation systems. Such systems include real environment-integrated games. Through these games, motor responses and desired movements are obtained from patients. The actual environments developed for the system are shown on the computer screen, virtual reality glasses, and tactile feedback devices. Physiotherapists can carry out both training and evaluation with this game-based method. Among telerehabilitation methods, the virtual reality method delivers active participation chances and motivates individuals [11].

4.3 Web-Based Approach in Telerehabilitation

There are web-based platforms for assessment, training, and exercise treatments with telerehabilitation methods in neurological patients. MyRehabPro, RehabPal, Longgood, RehabMypatient, and MOTMI are the leading platforms. These platforms have numerous advantages, such as showing exercise training through video, having an understandable system for patients to understand quickly, and allowing videoconferencing. The exercise training on these platforms is specific to pathology and involves many exercises, such as strengthening, stretching, balance, and breathing. Although these platforms had been used before the pandemic, they were primarily used during the pandemic period [12–14]. Among these platforms, exercise training and assessments are involved in the Longgood platform. The Motmi platform includes more neurological rehabilitation interventions compared to other rehabilitation areas.

4.4 Virtual Reality Approach in Telerehabilitation

Virtual reality can be defined as creating interactive simulations using computers, software, and additional devices, allowing individuals to feel as if they are in another environment and interact with that environment through body movement [15]. Traditional telerehabilitation systems do not incorporate virtual reality methods. The utilization of virtual reality in rehabilitation programs is increasingly on the rise. Virtual reality effectively creates environments, scenarios, and conditions conducive to daily life, aiming to facilitate an individual's adaptation to the advantages and disadvantages of the real-life environment. The benefits of telerehabilitation are enhanced by adding sensorimotor, cognitive, and social components through virtual reality. Virtual reality-based telerehabilitation simultaneously increases patient compliance with treatment by creating an enjoyable environment.

4.5 Telerehabilitation Principles in Neurological Rehabilitation

The principles of telerehabilitation in neurological diseases include rules, as in other diseases. Without an adequate cognitive level for neurological patients' consent and permission, which must be realized within an ethical and legal framework, written consent must be obtained from the patient's relatives, and patient's privacy must be given priority. The physiotherapist who will perform evaluation, treatment, and follow-up using the telerehabilitation method should have adequate knowledge about this web-based technological system, the patient, and the patient's pathology evaluation and treatment. Moreover, the physiotherapist should have communicative strength due to the disadvantage of not being in the same environment as the patient. Since telerehabilitation is teamwork, the physiotherapist should have solid and constant communication with the patient and other health and technical professionals in the team. Poor communication, inadequate technological infrastructure, and a lack of equipment and experience are among the factors that weaken the telerehabilitation process [7, 16]. Hence, patients' and their relatives' education, sociocultural, and economic levels must be considered. Since it is a neurological group, their mobility, balance, falls, and functionality must be thoroughly evaluated before rehabilitation and training, and a treatment plan should be drawn up without causing risk factors such as injury. It should be determined and explained to patients which method is more suitable for the telerehabilitation interventions and its purpose before the treatment. Patients and their relatives should be informed before the intervention, and trial applications should be carried out. The setting where telerehabilitation will be applied should be checked, and it should be decided whether the setting is suitable.

4.6 Telerehabilitation and Neuroplasticity

Neuroplasticity is the ability of the central nervous system to undergo structural changes in function and connections as a result of external or internal stimuli [17–19]. Neurological disorders affecting the brain disrupt an individual's communication with the external world [20]. Studies indicate that task-oriented and repetitive exercises are critical components in synaptic formation, especially following a stroke [21, 22]. Moreover, environmental enrichment is believed to impact neuroplasticity [23]. Telerehabilitation has been demonstrated to affect dynamic, spontaneous neural activity in multiple regions of the brain [24]. Telerehabilitation methods, particularly those creating a natural environment experience such as virtual reality technology, enable the repetitive and effective practice of motor skills in an enriched environment. Huang et al. [25] has shown that VR-supported telerehabilitation effectively increases Brain-Derived Neurotrophic Factor (BDNF), indicating neural connectivity formation in individuals with chronic stroke. VR applications implemented in individuals with stroke contribute to neuroplasticity with positive effects such as enhanced interhemispheric balance, increased cortical connectivity, heightened frontal lobe activation, transcranial magnetic stimulation expansion, and involvement of the mirror neuron system [18]. Telerehabilitation methods inherently containing increased feedback are believed to be effective in functional recovery, triggering neural plasticity components with the stimulation of sensory, cognitive, and perceptual-motor pathways [26].

4.7 Telerehabilitation and Task-Oriented Approach in Neurologic Rehabilitation

The task-oriented approach in neurorehabilitation is based on the principles of motor learning. For task-oriented training to be practical in individuals with neurological disorders, specific components of the exercises must be provided to trigger motor learning and neuroplasticity; these include being specific to real-world situations and content, being randomly sequenced, incorporating high and clustered repetitions, and aiming to restructure the entire task [21].

The number of studies combining a task-oriented approach with telerehabilitation in neurological disorders is limited in the literature. When we examine three studies integrating task-oriented training into telerehabilitation, in two studies, specific activities were divided into steps according to patients' disabilities and restricted movements and repeatedly provided through mobile applications [27, 28].

In the other study, a training system was provided in the form of stations, with different upper extremity activities at each station, and this was implemented in a videoconference format [29].

4.8 Motor Control and Telerehabilitation

Motor control ensures the control of the target-oriented movement at the level of the central nervous system and the correct perception of the movement with afferent and efferent pathways. It regulates the necessary mechanisms for performing the movement. Motor control is enabled by motor (movement), sensory (perceptual), and cognitive systems. Motor control should be integrated into treatments with the necessary neurophysiological approaches in telerehabilitation interventions, especially neurological rehabilitation. Motor control-based approaches should be adopted in telerehabilitation interventions for movement disorders, balance and coordination problems, and tonus problems. Motor control-based interventions are applied in many neurological rehabilitation interventions such as stroke, multiple sclerosis (MS), Parkinson's disease, and traumatic brain injuries (TBIs) [9–11, 14]. Owing to motor control, motor improvements are observed after a neurological pathology, and functionality and active participation of the patient in activities of daily living increase. Performing motor control-based exercises in patients with neurological deficits and complications facilitates neuroplasticity since neuroplasticity accelerates motor recovery. Neuroplasticity is important for motor control [12, 13]. Motor control-based exercises are thought to be more effective, particularly in individuals who have had a stroke. Motor control tends to regain the activity lost in the central nervous system and improves neuroplasticity [12, 13]. Virtual reality applications, especially among the telerehabilitation methods, include motor control-based approaches. Recent studies in the literature have indicated that there have been improvements in upper extremity function in individuals with stroke through virtual reality applications, and the improvements, as mentioned earlier, are based on motor control and neuroplasticity mechanisms [16, 30]. The virtual reality method of telerehabilitation interventions applied to neurological diseases is a motor control-based approach that enhances motor recovery in patients, improves functional capacity, and helps patients take an active role in daily life.

4.9 Multiple Sclerosis and Telerehabilitation

Multiple sclerosis is a neurodegenerative disease that most commonly causes disability in young adults worldwide [31]. The pathophysiology of MS involves axonal degeneration, brain atrophy, and autoimmune processes [32, 33]. Its symptoms manifest in a wide range, with the most common ones being walking and balance difficulties, sensory loss, pain, spasticity, fatigue, and urinary and sexual dysfunctions [34]. The majority of individuals diagnosed with MS are women and young adults [35–37]. Due to the age range of 20–30 years at the time of diagnosis and their active involvement in daily life and work, the participation rate in physiotherapy sessions in clinical settings can be low. In this context, telerehabilitation methods provide a significant advantage in the treatment of individuals with MS.

The most commonly used telerehabilitation methods in MS rehabilitation include video recordings, videoconferences, slides, mobile phone applications, games, and VR technologies. VR applications stand out mainly due to their included motor and cognitive components. Ortiz-Gutierrez et al. [38] stated a telerehabilitation method involving VR with Xbox and Kinect consoles was applied to individuals with MS for 10 weeks, with 4 sessions/week. As a result, the intervention group improved sensory processing skills, a crucial component in achieving balance and postural control. In another research, a 12-week telerehabilitation program is effective in the treatment of cognitive dysfunction, which is observed in more than half of individuals with MS [39–41].

Telerehabilitation can also be enriched by incorporating different methods such as motor imagery [42]. A study conducted by Shaw et al. [43] demonstrates that despite living in urban environments, receiving physiotherapy in a clinical setting imposes significant time and financial costs on individuals with MS. In studies, telerehabilitation and conventional physiotherapy methods have been observed to yield similar results in terms of functional outcome measures. Therefore, telerehabilitation can be preferred over face-to-face physiotherapy in a clinical setting.

In 2015, Amatya et al. [1] analyzed 12 studies investigating the effects of telerehabilitation on individuals with MS. They could not obtain a definitive conclusion due to the insufficient methodological quality and quantity of the studies. With the widespread adoption of telerehabilitation applications during the COVID-19 pandemic in 2020, the number of high-quality studies on this topic has also increased.

4.10 Parkinson's Disease and Telerehabilitation

Parkinson's disease is the second most commonly encountered neurodegenerative disease worldwide [44]. Symptoms such as bradykinesia, tremor, postural instability, and rigidity are frequently associated with Parkinson's [45]. Another characteristic feature of Parkinson's disease is the Freezing of Gait (FoG) [46].

In the majority of the studies in the literature, telerehabilitation and virtual reality applications have been examined separately. To utilize telerehabilitation methods, cognitive functions must be preserved in this group of patients. This level has been implemented as a minimum of 24 points on the Mini Mental Score Examination (MMSE) in studies.

Vellata et al. [47] compiled the results of studies conducted on 421 individuals with Parkinson's disease by reviewing 15 articles, forming a systematic review. The results of this systematic review indicate that telerehabilitation is effective in maintaining or improving components such as walking, balance, quality of life, speech and voice, and patient satisfaction [47]. In individuals with Parkinson's disease, if we look at the effects of exergaming, smartwatches, consoles, or mobile applications on motor functions in two studies, it is more effective than conventional physiotherapy in improving quality of life (QOL) and participation rates. However, the two treatments have yet to demonstrate superiority over each other in parameters such as disease severity or balance [48].

According to the literature, the duration of telerehabilitation studies aiming to improve motor functions in Parkinson's disease varies between 5 and 16 weeks. When examining the content of telerehabilitation applications, it is observed that the weekly session frequency ranges between 2 and 3 sessions, with session durations varying between 30 and 50 min. When interpreting the effects of telerehabilitation on individuals with Parkinson's disease, it should be noted that in most studies, treatments were applied to groups consisting of physically independent individuals with Hoehn & Yahr scores of 3 and below. To assess the effects of telerehabilitation for individuals with Parkinson's disease who have a severe disability or rely on a wheelchair for mobility, studies including this group of patients are needed.

4.11 Spinal Cord Injuries and Telerehabilitation

After spinal cord injuries (SCIs), the health condition of individuals is worse than that of healthy individuals. Therefore, functionality is severely affected, and quality of life is reduced. Thus, living after a spinal cord injury involves a complicated process [49, 50]. Individuals with SCI experience limitations on independence and incompetence in self-care activities. The difficulties above are usually the activities that require special care in the daily life process [10, 11]. Hence, telehealth interventions are an essential service for individuals with SCI.

Telerehabilitation is known to provide positive effects on individuals with SCI, and individuals have a positive attitude toward this intervention. It is known that studies on this subject have resulted in significant improvements in emotional states, quality of life, functionality, tonus disorders, pain conditions, and even bladder-gut dysfunction [51–54].

In individuals with SCI, telerehabilitation ensures strong communication between the patient and the healthcare professional, in addition to its effects on complications and treatment, supports clinical adherence, increases the patient's motivation, ensures that the healthcare professional sees the patient's home setting, makes arrangements, and observes the situations that may pose a risk or interfere with the patient's functionality [55].

Re-hospitalizations are standard in individuals with spinal cord injuries. Telerehabilitation and telehealth methods show that hospitalization frequencies are reduced or even prevented as diseases and complications are controlled. Therefore, telehealth interventions are beneficial regarding transportation and hospital costs [3, 51, 56]. Re-hospitalization has significant benefits in terms of cost and the success of rehabilitation and prevention of complications.

Only some patients with spinal cord injury are eligible for telerehabilitation. Telerehabilitation is less effective in individuals who live outside the city center, have accessibility problems, or cannot afford the necessary equipment and Internet infrastructure for this health model and who instead need physical evaluation and manual treatment due to the functionally affected upper extremity, except the sacral region, and trunk muscles. Especially for all functional levels, the acute period is not preferred as an appropriate time for telerehabilitation. Telerehabilitation intervention in individuals with SCI should be well-decided according to the patient, functionality status, home setting, time of injury, length of hospital stay, easy access status, and most importantly, the patient's preference [57–62].

Although telerehabilitation in neurological diseases has been very popular in recent years, the use of telerehabilitation in patients with spinal cord injuries has fallen behind other diseases [51, 59]. It is thought that patients with spinal cord injury prefer this method less because they have more disability and loss of mobility and function [63, 64].

In summary, telerehabilitation and telehealth interventions in SCI patients are adequate for ensuring functionality, which requires special care in daily life, for reducing the cost of clinical support, for more active participation of the patient in daily life, and treatment according to the level of functionality [65].

4.12 Stroke and Telerehabilitation

Stroke is ranked among the top three pathologies worldwide that lead to death and severe disability [66, 67]. Individuals poststroke encounter numerous motor and non-motor symptoms, including muscle weakness, spasticity, balance impairment, falls, limitations in activities of daily living, loss of fine motor skills in the upper extremities, and symptoms such as depression [68, 69]. These symptoms significantly and negatively impact the quality of life of individuals [70–72].

In the literature, a high session adherence rate (>80%) has been observed in the majority of studies implementing telerehabilitation in individuals with stroke [73]. In examination of adverse effects, symptoms such as fatigue and upper extremity pain were encountered at a low rate. The literature includes numerous studies that have implemented telerehabilitation on individuals poststroke using various methods and have examined its effectiveness in different components. Regardless of the application method, telerehabilitation demonstrates high usability and satisfaction rates in individuals within this population [70, 71, 73, 74]. In general, telerehabilitation interventions administered to individuals with stroke yield similar results when compared to physiotherapy provided in clinical settings [75].

In a meta-analysis, it has been demonstrated that telerehabilitation is more effective than conventional methods in improving upper extremity motor functions [14]. When the details of telerehabilitation applications in individuals with stroke are examined, the application frequency varies from daily sessions to 3 sessions/week, and the application duration ranges from 10 days to 12 weeks. Supervision in telerehabilitation applications is implemented in various ways. Partial or full-time supervision can be provided through the telerehabilitation system, or it can be provided physically.

4.13 Intracranial Tumor and Telerehabilitation

Problems such as motor, sensory, and cognitive disorders are frequently observed after intracranial tumor surgeries. These problems affect the participation of patients in daily life and reduce their functionality and quality of life [76, 77]. Cognitive disorders, which should be attached to treatment for motor and sensory disorders, substantially reduce the adaptation to rehabilitation and participation in treatment [78]. Cognitive rehabilitation should be given priority to minimize these effects caused by the mental state. Studies have recently shown cognitive rehabilitation benefits patients undergoing intracranial tumor surgery [79–81]. Since cognitive rehabilitation interventions are still not carried out in every clinic nowadays and transportation is difficult and costly in clinics where it is carried out, access is not as easy as routine rehabilitation. This situation causes severe problems in terms of the treatment status of patient [82, 83]. Based on the limitations of these problems and traditional methods, cognitive rehabilitation is also addressed with telerehabilitation interventions, which are popular and advantageous nowadays. These clinical pictures in telerehabilitation interventions, especially virtual reality methods, are known to positively affect adaptation to treatment, participation, motivation, and recovery of the patient and have positive emotional effects [7]. In patients who have undergone intracranial tumor surgery, telerehabilitation is realized through not only cognitive symptoms but also motor and sensory symptoms. Using virtual reality, video-based applications, and teleconferencing methods, appropriate treatments such as upper and lower extremity and trunk muscle strengthening training, balance training, and normal joint range of motion exercises can be performed for motor symptoms. With this method, even in-home arrangements can be made for balance problems and falling problems caused by muscle weakness of the individual. For sensory symptoms, sensory training that the individual can do on their own can be provided. Even before undergoing intracranial tumor surgery, patients are trained in treatment, evaluation, and telerehabilitation methods in the preoperative period. Telerehabilitation interventions can be performed after surgery and for symptoms that may arise before surgery and patient-family education. Problems involving face-to-face treatment, controlling the patient, lack of communication, fall possibilities, and web-based accessibility problems, among the disadvantages of telerehabilitation, also apply to intracranial patients.

4.14 Pediatric Neurological Diseases and Telerehabilitation

Technology-based interventions are gaining importance for rehabilitating neurologically affected children [84]. Telerehabilitation interventions can be performed with game-based applications for numerous pathologies such as cerebral palsy, brachial plexus, muscle diseases, and spina bifida. In pediatric patients, motor and sensory training can be provided, primarily through game-based activities of virtual reality applications. In pediatric patients, these interventions address both motor and sensory training and cognitive and behavioral problems. Recent studies in the literature have highlighted that telerehabilitation interventions can also improve mental and behavioral domains in pediatric neurological patients [85–87]. Telerehabilitation is extremely important for pediatric patients regarding access to cognitive rehabilitation, transportation, and cost, particularly for adult neurological patients.

Telerehabilitation has ensured elaborate follow-up and performance in pediatric patients [87]. Telerehabilitation involves follow-up, evaluation, and treatment processes in affected pediatric patients. Web-based telerehabilitation applications allow healthcare professionals to perform daily interventions and manage settings. To ensure motor and sensory integration, they determine game-based exercises and activities, adjust the difficulty levels of these exercises and activities in the following days, and add new activities. These exercises and activities increase the child's success and motivation. In these activities and exercises, interventions can also be made through Internet access and software. These interventions provide important feedback for the child and healthcare professionals [88–92].

Furthermore, in pediatric patients, telerehabilitation interventions are applied not only for functionality but also for dyslexia, attention deficit, and hyperactivity disorder [93, 94]. Attention should be paid to specific issues regarding telerehabilitation interventions in pediatric and adult patients. There are numerous factors such as parental consent, adequate sociocultural and communication level of the parent, providing the necessary equipment, and the presence of the infrastructure systems required. Before interventions, it is recommended to provide family education and, if necessary, to have face-to-face interviews with the family. The setting where the intervention will be carried out and the arrangements at home should be checked (Fig. 4.1).

Fig. 4.1 Positive effects of telerehabilitation in neurological disorders

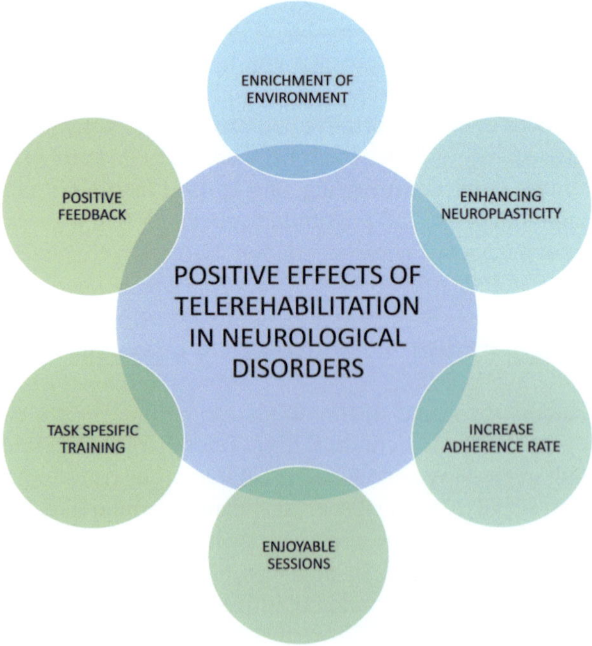

References

1. Amatya B, Galea MP, Kesselring J, Khan F. Effectiveness of telerehabilitation interventions in persons with multiple sclerosis: a systematic review. Mult Scler Relat Disord. 2015;4(4):358–69. https://doi.org/10.1016/j.msard.2015.06.011.
2. Appleby E, Gill ST, Hayes LK, Walker TL, Walsh M, Kumar S. Effectiveness of telerehabilitation in the management of adults with stroke: a systematic review. PLoS One. 2019;14(11):e0225150. https://doi.org/10.1371/journal.pone.0225150.
3. Irgens I, Rekand T, Arora M, Liu N, Marshall R, Biering-Sørensen F, et al. Telehealth for people with spinal cord injury: a narrative review. Spinal Cord. 2018;56(7):643–55. https://doi.org/10.1038/s41393-017-0033-3.
4. Shem K, Irgens I, Alexander M. Getting started: mechanisms of telerehabilitation. In: Telerehabilitation. Elsevier; 2022. p. 5–20.
5. Forman CR, Nielsen JB, Lorentzen J. Neuroplasticity at home: improving home-based motor learning through technological solutions. A review. Front Rehabil Sci. 2021;2:789165. https://doi.org/10.3389/fresc.2021.789165.
6. Levin MF, Weiss PL, Keshner EA. Emergence of virtual reality as a tool for upper limb rehabilitation: incorporation of motor control and motor learning principles. Phys Ther. 2015;95(3):415–25. https://doi.org/10.2522/ptj.20130579.
7. Torrisi M, Maresca G, De Cola MC, Cannavò A, Sciarrone F, Silvestri G, et al. Using telerehabilitation to improve cognitive function in post-stroke survivors: is this the time for the continuity of care? Int J Rehabil Res. 2019;42(4):344–51.
8. Fiani B, Siddiqi I, Lee SC, Dhillon L. Telerehabilitation: development, application, and need for increased usage in the COVID-19 era for patients with spinal pathology. Cureus. 2020;12(9):e10563. https://doi.org/10.7759/cureus.10563.
9. Malik AN, Tariq H, Afridi A, Rathore FA. Technological advancements in stroke rehabilitation. J Pak Med Assoc. 2022;72:1672–4.
10. Klamroth-Marganska V. Stroke rehabilitation: therapy robots and assistive devices. Adv Exp Med Biol. 2018;1065:579–87.
11. Choi Y-H, Paik N-J. Mobile game-based virtual reality program for upper extremity stroke rehabilitation. J Vis Exp. 2018;133:56241. https://doi.org/10.3791/56241.
12. Chen AI, Xiong L-J, Tong YU, Mao M. The neuroprotective roles of BDNF in hypoxic ischemic brain injury. Biomed Rep. 2013;1(2):167–76. https://doi.org/10.3892/br.2012.48.
13. Pin-Barre C, Laurin J. Physical exercise as a diagnostic, rehabilitation, and preventive tool: influence on neuroplasticity and motor recovery after stroke. Neural Plast. 2015;2015:1–12. https://doi.org/10.1155/2015/608581.
14. Doumas I, Everard G, Dehem S, Lejeune T. Serious games for upper limb rehabilitation after stroke: a meta-analysis. J NeuroEng Rehabil. 2021;18(1):100. https://doi.org/10.1186/s12984-021-00889-1.
15. Wohlgenannt I, Simons A, Stieglitz S. Virtual reality. Bus Inf Syst Eng. 2020;62:455–61.
16. Song Y-H, Lee H-M. Effect of immersive virtual reality-based bilateral arm training in patients with chronic stroke. Brain Sci. 2021;11(8):1032. https://doi.org/10.3390/brainsci11081032.
17. Grafman J. Conceptualizing functional neuroplasticity. J Commun Disord. 2000;33(4):345–56. https://doi.org/10.1016/S0021-9924(00)00030-7.
18. Cheung KL, Tunik E, Adamovich SV, Boyd LA. Neuroplasticity and virtual reality. In: Virtual reality for physical and motor rehabilitation. Springer; 2014. p. 5–24.
19. Cramer SC, Sur M, Dobkin BH, O'Brien C, Sanger TD, Trojanowski JQ, et al. Harnessing neuroplasticity for clinical applications. Brain. 2011;34:1591–609.
20. Kitzmüller G, Häggström T, Asplund K. Living an unfamiliar body: the significance of the long-term influence of bodily changes on the perception of self after stroke. Med Health Care Philos. 2013;16:19–29.
21. Harvey RL. Improving poststroke recovery: neuroplasticity and task-oriented training. Curr Treat Options Cardiovasc Med. 2009;11(3):251–9. https://doi.org/10.1007/s11936-009-0026-4.

22. Rungseethanakul S, Tretriluxana J, Piriyaprasarth P, Pakaprot N, Jitaree K, Tretriluxana S, et al. Task oriented training activities post stroke will produce measurable alterations in brain plasticity concurrent with skill improvement. Top Stroke Rehabil. 2022;29(4):241–54.
23. Neves LT, Paz LV, Wieck A, Mestriner RG, de Miranda Monteiro VAC, Xavier LL. Environmental enrichment in stroke research: an update. Transl Stroke Res. 2024;15(2):339–51. https://doi.org/10.1007/s12975-023-01132-w.
24. Chen J, Li J, Qiao F, Shi Z, Lu W. Effects of home-based telerehabilitation on dynamic alterations in regional intrinsic neural activity and degree centrality in stroke patients. PeerJ. 2023;11:e15903. https://doi.org/10.7717/peerj.15903.
25. Huang C-Y, Chiang W-C, Yeh Y-C, Fan S-C, Yang W-H, Kuo H-C, et al. Effects of virtual reality-based motor control training on inflammation, oxidative stress, neuroplasticity and upper limb motor function in patients with chronic stroke: a randomized controlled trial. BMC Neurol. 2022;22(1):21. https://doi.org/10.1186/s12883-021-02547-4.
26. Hao J, Xie H, Harp K, Chen Z, Siu K-C. Effects of virtual reality intervention on neural plasticity in stroke rehabilitation: a systematic review. Arch Phys Med Rehabil. 2022;103(3):523–41. https://doi.org/10.1016/j.apmr.2021.06.024.
27. Eldemir S, Guclu-Gunduz A, Eldemir K, Saygili F, Yilmaz R, Akbostancı MC. The effect of task-oriented circuit training-based telerehabilitation on upper extremity motor functions in patients with Parkinson's disease: a randomized controlled trial. Parkinsonism Relat Disord. 2023;109:105334. https://doi.org/10.1016/j.parkreldis.2023.105334.
28. Doğan M, Ayvat E, Kılınç M. Telerehabilitation versus virtual reality supported task-oriented circuit therapy on upper limbs and trunk functions in patients with multiple sclerosis: a randomized controlled study. Mult Scler Relat Disord. 2023;71:104558.
29. Lin C-C, Lin Y-C, Hsu H-Y, Lin Y-S, Su F-C, Kuo L-C. Home-based tele-rehabilitation system provides task-oriented training courses based on the stages of stroke. In: 2021 IEEE Region 10 Symposium (TENSYMP). IEEE; 2021. p. 1–5.
30. ÖGÜN MN, Kurul R, YaŞAr MF, Turkoglu SA, Avci Ş, Yildiz N. Effect of leap motion-based 3D immersive virtual reality usage on upper extremity function in ischemic stroke patients. Arq Neuropsiquiatr. 2019;77(10):681–8. https://doi.org/10.1590/0004-282x20190129.
31. Dobson R, Giovannoni G. Multiple sclerosis—a review. Eur J Neurol. 2019;26:27–40.
32. Korn T. Pathophysiology of multiple sclerosis. J Neurol. 2008;255(S6):2–6. https://doi.org/10.1007/s00415-008-6001-2.
33. Zéphir H. Progress in understanding the pathophysiology of multiple sclerosis. Rev Neurol. 2018;174(6):358–63. https://doi.org/10.1016/j.neurol.2018.03.006.
34. Lublin FD. Clinical features and diagnosis of multiple sclerosis. Neurol Clin. 2005;23(1):1–15. https://doi.org/10.1016/j.ncl.2004.09.003.
35. Sellner J, Kraus J, Awad A, Milo R, Hemmer B, Stüve O. The increasing incidence and prevalence of female multiple sclerosis—a critical analysis of potential environmental factors. Autoimmun Rev. 2011;10(8):495–502. https://doi.org/10.1016/j.autrev.2011.02.006.
36. McGinley MP, Goldschmidt CH, Rae-Grant AD. Diagnosis and treatment of multiple sclerosis. JAMA. 2021;325(8):765. https://doi.org/10.1001/jama.2020.26858.
37. Ford H. Clinical presentation and diagnosis of multiple sclerosis. Clin Med. 2020;20(4):380–3. https://doi.org/10.7861/clinmed.2020-0292.
38. Ortiz-Gutiérrez R, Cano-de-la-Cuerda R, Galán-del-Río F, Alguacil-Diego I, Palacios-Ceña D, Miangolarra-Page J. A telerehabilitation program improves postural control in multiple sclerosis patients: a Spanish preliminary study. Int J Environ Res Public Health. 2013;10(11):5697–710. https://doi.org/10.3390/ijerph10115697.
39. Charvet LE, Yang J, Shaw MT, Sherman K, Haider L, Xu J, et al. Cognitive function in multiple sclerosis improves with telerehabilitation: results from a randomized controlled trial. PLoS One. 2017;12(5):e0177177. https://doi.org/10.1371/journal.pone.0177177.
40. Piras MR. Longitudinal study of cognitive dysfunction in multiple sclerosis: neuropsychological, neuroradiological, and neurophysiological findings. J Neurol Neurosurg Psychiatry. 2003;74(7):878–85. https://doi.org/10.1136/jnnp.74.7.878.

41. Chiaravalloti ND, DeLuca J. Cognitive impairment in multiple sclerosis. Lancet Neurol. 2008;7(12):1139–51. https://doi.org/10.1016/S1474-4422(08)70259-X.
42. Kahraman T, Savci S, Ozdogar AT, Gedik Z, Idiman E. Physical, cognitive and psychosocial effects of telerehabilitation-based motor imagery training in people with multiple sclerosis: a randomized controlled pilot trial. J Telemed Telecare. 2020;26(5):251–60. https://doi.org/10.1177/1357633X18822355.
43. Shaw MT, Best P, Frontario A, Charvet LE. Telerehabilitation benefits patients with multiple sclerosis in an urban setting. J Telemed Telecare. 2021;27(1):39–45. https://doi.org/10.1177/1357633X19861830.
44. Jankovic J. Parkinson's disease: clinical features and diagnosis. J Neurol Neurosurg Psychiatry. 2008;79(4):368–76. https://doi.org/10.1136/jnnp.2007.131045.
45. Lee A, Gilbert RM. Epidemiology of Parkinson disease. Neurol Clin. 2016;34(4):955–65. https://doi.org/10.1016/j.ncl.2016.06.012.
46. Okuma Y. Freezing of gait in Parkinson's disease. J Neurol. 2006;253(S7):vii27–32. https://doi.org/10.1007/s00415-006-7007-2.
47. Vellata C, Belli S, Balsamo F, Giordano A, Colombo R, Maggioni G. Effectiveness of telerehabilitation on motor impairments, non-motor symptoms and compliance in patients with Parkinson's disease: a systematic review. Front Neurol. 2021;12:627999. https://doi.org/10.3389/fneur.2021.627999.
48. Özden F. The effect of mobile application-based rehabilitation in patients with Parkinson's disease: a systematic review and meta-analysis. Clin Neurol Neurosurg. 2023;225:107579. https://doi.org/10.1016/j.clineuro.2022.107579.
49. Biering-Sørensen F, Bickenbach JE, El Masry WS, Officer A, von Groote PM. ISCoS–WHO collaboration. International Perspectives of Spinal Cord Injury (IPSCI) report. Spinal Cord. 2011;49(6):679–83. https://doi.org/10.1038/sc.2011.12.
50. Middleton A, Downer B, Haas A, Knox S, Ottenbacher KJ. Functional status is associated with 30-day potentially preventable readmissions following home health care. Med Care. 2019;57(2):145–51. https://doi.org/10.1097/MLR.0000000000001047.
51. Lee S, Kim J, Kim J. Substantiating clinical effectiveness and potential barriers to the widespread implementation of spinal cord injury telerehabilitation: a systematic review and qualitative synthesis of randomized trials in the recent past decade. Telemed Rep. 2021;2(1):64–77.
52. Coulter EH, McLean AN, Hasler JP, Allan DB, McFadyen A, Paul L. The effectiveness and satisfaction of web-based physiotherapy in people with spinal cord injury: a pilot randomised controlled trial. Spinal Cord. 2017;55(4):383–9. https://doi.org/10.1038/sc.2016.125.
53. Sechrist S, Lavoie S, Khong C-M, Dirlikov B, Shem K. Telemedicine using an iPad in the spinal cord injury population: a utility and patient satisfaction study. Spinal Cord Ser Cases. 2018;4(1):71. https://doi.org/10.1038/s41394-018-0105-4.
54. Al-Taleb MKH, Purcell M, Fraser M, Petric-Gray N, Vuckovic A. Home used, patient self-managed, brain-computer interface for the management of central neuropathic pain post spinal cord injury: usability study. J NeuroEng Rehabil. 2019;16(1):128. https://doi.org/10.1186/s12984-019-0588-7.
55. Zulman DM, Verghese A. Virtual care, telemedicine visits, and real connection in the era of COVID-19. JAMA. 2021;325(5):437. https://doi.org/10.1001/jama.2020.27304.
56. Woo C, Guihan M, Frick C, Gill CM, Ho CH. What's happening now! Telehealth management of spinal cord injury/disorders. J Spinal Cord Med. 2011;34(3):322–31. https://doi.org/10.1179/2045772311Y.0000000003.
57. Ho C, Atchison K, Noonan VK, McKenzie N, Cadel L, Ganshorn H, et al. Models of care delivery from rehabilitation to community for spinal cord injury: a scoping review. J Neurotrauma. 2021;38(6):677–97. https://doi.org/10.1089/neu.2020.7396.
58. Hamilton R, Driver S, Noorani S, Callender L, Bennett M, Monden K. Utilization and access to healthcare services among community-dwelling people living with spinal cord injury. J Spinal Cord Med. 2017;40(3):321–8.

59. Hatch MN, Martinez RN, Etingen B, Cotner B, Hogan TP, Wickremasinghe IM, et al. Characterization of telehealth use in veterans with spinal cord injuries and disorders. PM R. 2021;13(10):1094–103. https://doi.org/10.1002/pmrj.12515.
60. Walia S, Wolfe D, Keast D, Ho C, Ethans K, Worley S, et al. Facilitators and barriers for implementing an internet clinic for the treatment of pressure injuries. Telemed eHealth. 2019;25(12):1237–43.
61. Tung JY, Stead B, Mann W, Pham B, Popovic MR. Assistive technologies for self-managed pressure ulcer prevention in spinal cord injury: a scoping review. J Rehabil Res Dev. 2015;52(2):131–46. https://doi.org/10.1682/JRRD.2014.02.0064.
62. Gustafson K, Stillman M, Capron M, O'Connell C, Longoni Di Giusto M, Tyagi N, et al. COVID-19 and spinal cord injury and disease: results of an international survey as the pandemic progresses. Spinal Cord Ser Cases. 2021;7(1):13. https://doi.org/10.1038/s41394-020-00356-4.
63. Dobransky K, Hargittai E. Unrealized potential: exploring the digital disability divide. Poetics. 2016;58:18–28.
64. Duplaga M. Digital divide among people with disabilities: analysis of data from a nationwide study for determinants of Internet use and activities performed online. PLoS One. 2017;12(6):e0179825. https://doi.org/10.1371/journal.pone.0179825.
65. Kryger MA, Crytzer TM, Fairman A, Quinby EJ, Karavolis M, Pramana G, et al. The effect of the interactive mobile health and rehabilitation system on health and psychosocial outcomes in spinal cord injury: randomized controlled trial. J Med Internet Res. 2019;21(8):e14305. https://doi.org/10.2196/14305.
66. Katan M, Luft A. Global burden of stroke. Semin Neurol. 2018;38(02):208–11. https://doi.org/10.1055/s-0038-1649503.
67. Mukherjee D, Patil CG. Epidemiology and the global burden of stroke. World Neurosurg. 2011;76(6):S85–90. https://doi.org/10.1016/j.wneu.2011.07.023.
68. Beyaert C, Vasa R, Frykberg GE. Gait post-stroke: pathophysiology and rehabilitation strategies. Clin Neurophysiol. 2015;45(4–5):335–55. https://doi.org/10.1016/j.neucli.2015.09.005.
69. Handelzalts S, Melzer I, Soroker N. Analysis of brain lesion impact on balance and gait following stroke. Front Hum Neurosci. 2019;13:149. https://doi.org/10.3389/fnhum.2019.00149.
70. Ramos-Lima MJM, Brasileiro IC, de Lima TL, Braga-Neto P. Quality of life after stroke: impact of clinical and sociodemographic factors. Clinics. 2018;73:e418. https://doi.org/10.6061/clinics/2017/e418.
71. Nichols-Larsen DS, Clark PC, Zeringue A, Greenspan A, Blanton S. Factors influencing stroke survivors' quality of life during subacute recovery. Stroke. 2005;36(7):1480–4. https://doi.org/10.1161/01.STR.0000170706.13595.4f.
72. Jeon NE, Kwon KM, Kim YH, Lee JS. The factors associated with health-related quality of life in stroke survivors age 40 and older. Ann Rehabil Med. 2017;41(5):743. https://doi.org/10.5535/arm.2017.41.5.743.
73. Stephenson A, Howes S, Murphy PJ, Deutsch JE, Stokes M, Pedlow K, et al. Factors influencing the delivery of telerehabilitation for stroke: a systematic review. PLoS One. 2022;17(5):e0265828. https://doi.org/10.1371/journal.pone.0265828.
74. Piron L, Turolla A, Tonin P, Piccione F, Lain L, Dam M. Satisfaction with care in post-stroke patients undergoing a telerehabilitation programme at home. J Telemed Telecare. 2008;14(5):257–60. https://doi.org/10.1258/jtt.2008.080304.
75. Chen J, Jin W, Zhang X-X, Xu W, Liu X-N, Ren C-C. Telerehabilitation approaches for stroke patients: systematic review and meta-analysis of randomized controlled trials. J Stroke Cerebrovasc Dis. 2015;24(12):2660–8. https://doi.org/10.1016/j.jstrokecerebrovasdis.2015.09.014.
76. Aaronson NK, Taphoorn MJB, Heimans JJ, Postma TJ, Gundy CM, Beute GN, et al. Compromised health-related quality of life in patients with low-grade glioma. J Clin Oncol. 2011;29(33):4430–5. https://doi.org/10.1200/JCO.2011.35.5750.
77. Waagemans ML, van Nieuwenhuizen D, Dijkstra M, Wumkes M, Dirven CMF, Leenstra S, et al. Long-term impact of cognitive deficits and epilepsy on quality of life in patients

with low-grade meningiomas. Neurosurgery. 2011;69(1):72–9. https://doi.org/10.1227/NEU.0b013e318212badb.
78. Cumming TB, Marshall RS, Lazar RM. Stroke, cognitive deficits, and rehabilitation: still an incomplete picture. Int J Stroke. 2013;8(1):38–45. https://doi.org/10.1111/j.1747-4949.2012.00972.x.
79. Gehring K, Sitskoorn MM, Gundy CM, Sikkes SAM, Klein M, Postma TJ, et al. Cognitive rehabilitation in patients with gliomas: a randomized, controlled trial. J Clin Oncol. 2009;27(22):3712–22. https://doi.org/10.1200/JCO.2008.20.5765.
80. Zucchella C, Capone A, Codella V, De Nunzio AM, Vecchione C, Sandrini G, et al. Cognitive rehabilitation for early post-surgery inpatients affected by primary brain tumor: a randomized, controlled trial. J Neuro-Oncol. 2013;114(1):93–100. https://doi.org/10.1007/s11060-013-1153-z.
81. Maschio M, Dinapoli L, Fabi A, Giannarelli D, Cantelmi T. Cognitive rehabilitation training in patients with brain tumor-related epilepsy and cognitive deficits: a pilot study. J Neuro-Oncol. 2015;125(2):419–26. https://doi.org/10.1007/s11060-015-1933-8.
82. Pace A, Villani V, Parisi C, Di Felice S, Lamaro M, Falcicchio C, et al. Rehabilitation pathways in adult brain tumor patients in the first 12 months of disease. A retrospective analysis of services utilization in 719 patients. Support Care Cancer. 2016;24(11):4801–6. https://doi.org/10.1007/s00520-016-3333-9.
83. Langbecker D, Yates P. Primary brain tumor patients' supportive care needs and multidisciplinary rehabilitation, community and psychosocial support services: awareness, referral and utilization. J Neuro-Oncol. 2016;127(1):91–102. https://doi.org/10.1007/s11060-015-2013-9.
84. Corti C, Oldrati V, Oprandi MC, Ferrari E, Poggi G, Borgatti R, et al. Remote technology-based training programs for children with acquired brain injury: a systematic review and a meta-analytic exploration. Behav Neurol. 2019;2019:1–31. https://doi.org/10.1155/2019/1346987.
85. How T-V, Hwang AS, Green REA, Mihailidis A. Envisioning future cognitive telerehabilitation technologies: a co-design process with clinicians. Disabil Rehabil Assist Technol. 2017;12(3):244–61. https://doi.org/10.3109/17483107.2015.1129457.
86. Kueider AM, Parisi JM, Gross AL, Rebok GW. Computerized cognitive training with older adults: a systematic review. PLoS One. 2012;7(7):e40588. https://doi.org/10.1371/journal.pone.0040588.
87. Zampolini M, Ilsbroukx S, Macellari V. Tele-rehabilitation: present and future. Ann Ist Super Sanita. 2008;44(2):125–34.
88. Thorell LB, Lindqvist S, Bergman Nutley S, Bohlin G, Klingberg T. Training and transfer effects of executive functions in preschool children. Dev Sci. 2009;12(1):106–13. https://doi.org/10.1111/j.1467-7687.2008.00745.x.
89. Diamond A, Lee K. Interventions shown to aid executive function development in children 4 to 12 years old. Science. 2011;333(6045):959–64. https://doi.org/10.1126/science.1204529.
90. Chacko A, Uderman J, Feirsen N, Bedard A-C, Marks D. Learning and cognitive disorders. Child Adolesc Psychiatr Clin N Am. 2013;22(3):457–77. https://doi.org/10.1016/j.chc.2013.03.006.
91. Wexler J, Vaughn S, Edmonds M, Reutebuch CK. A synthesis of fluency interventions for secondary struggling readers. Read Writ. 2008;21(4):317–47. https://doi.org/10.1007/s11145-007-9085-7.
92. Klingberg T, Fernell E, Olesen PJ, Johnson M, Gustafsson P, Dahlström K, et al. Computerized training of working memory in children with ADHD—a randomized, controlled trial. J Am Acad Child Adolesc Psychiatry. 2005;44(2):177–86. https://doi.org/10.1097/00004583-200502000-00010.
93. Pecini C, Spoglianti S, Michetti S, Bonetti S, Di Lieto MC, Gasperini F, et al. Telerehabilitation in developmental dyslexia: methods of implementation and expected results. Minerva Pediatr. 2018;70(6):529–38. https://doi.org/10.23736/S0026-4946.16.04426-1.
94. Simone M, Viterbo RG, Margari L, Iaffaldano P. Computer-assisted rehabilitation of attention in pediatric multiple sclerosis and ADHD patients: a pilot trial. BMC Neurol. 2018;18(1):82. https://doi.org/10.1186/s12883-018-1087-3.

Teleassessment Methods in Cardiopulmonary Rehabilitation

5

Rıdvan Aktan and Hazal Yakut Ozdemir

5.1 Introduction

Pandemics in the world have led to the development of extraordinary solutions that go beyond the social routine. During the pandemic period, the capacity of the health system was exceeded, and new solutions were sought for the proper continuation of healthcare services with the developing technology. With the Coronavirus (COVID-19) pandemic, telehealth applications continue to progress toward becoming an alternative health service. Such remote methods have continued to increase during and after the COVID-19 pandemic [1]. No specific method is used for telehealth applications, and applications such as phone calls, messaging, e-mail or videoconferencing, artificial intelligence technologies, and/or web-based applications can transfer data [2, 3].

There are various barriers for patients to access center-based healthcare. These barriers may be due to the health system, health center, patient, or global events such as the pandemic (see Fig. 5.1). Telehealth and teleassessment methods have been proposed to minimize barriers to accessing healthcare [4]. Telehealth uses remote mental and physical healthcare to assess, prevent, and intervene. Teleassessment was defined as "diagnostic, psychological assessment procedures administered to (an) individual(s) who is not in the same room as the examiner through the use of telecommunication technologies" by Krach et al. [5]. Teleassessment methods are remote technology-mediated delivery of assessments designed to be administered face-to-face in center-based services [5]. Teleassessment methods serve individuals who cannot access health services and aim to overcome

R. Aktan
Izmir University of Economics, Izmir, Turkey

H. Yakut Ozdemir (✉)
Izmir Democracy University, Izmir, Turkey
e-mail: hazal.yakutozdemir@idu.edu.tr

F. Özden et al. (eds.), *Telerehabilitation*, TELe-Health,
https://doi.org/10.1007/978-3-031-69080-8_5

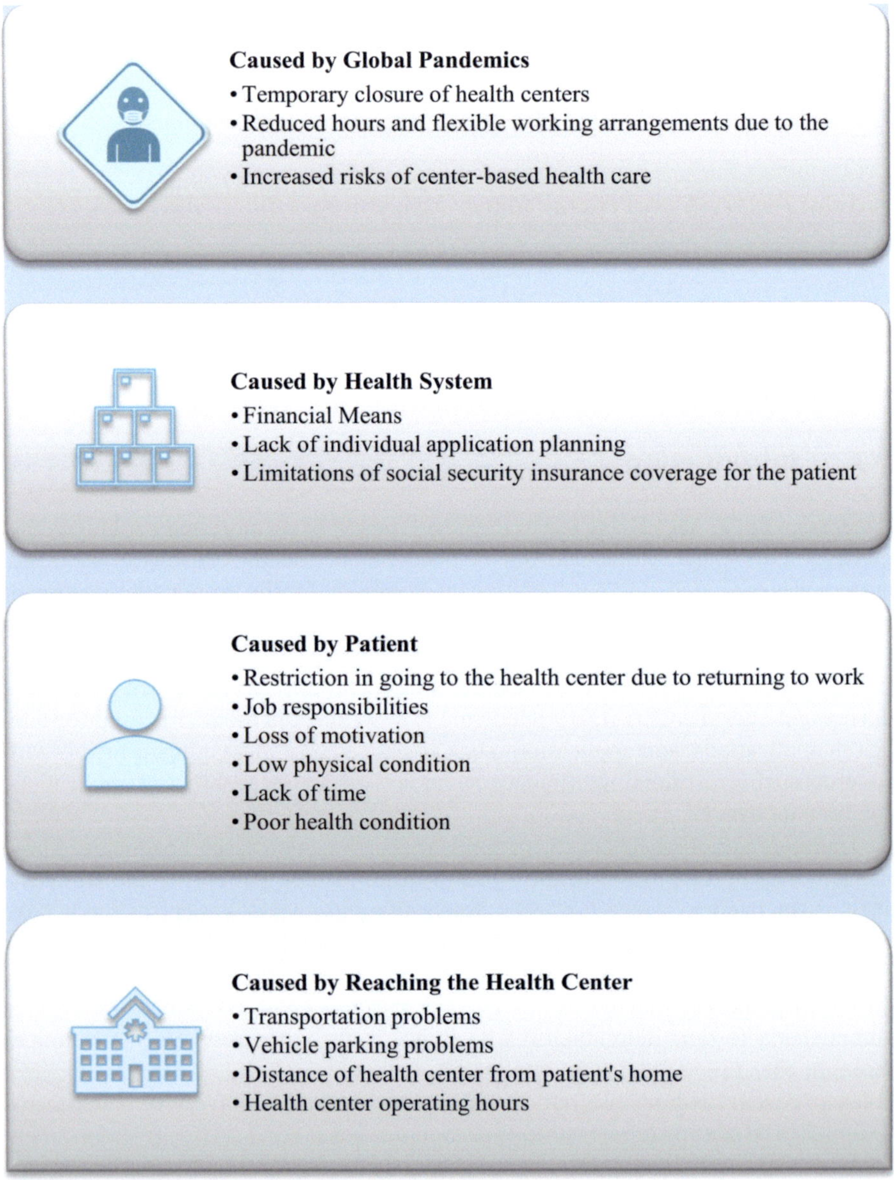

Fig. 5.1 Barriers to access to center-based health services

barriers to accessing services [3, 6]. These methods are also used for setting rehabilitation goals and evaluating the effectiveness of exercise and rehabilitation interventions in line with disease management in the cardiopulmonary field [7]. This chapter will scrutinize the literature's requirements, methods, and examples for tele-assessment in the cardiopulmonary rehabilitation field.

5.2 Cardiopulmonary Teleassessment and Technologies

Cardiopulmonary teleassessment can be synchronous or asynchronous, and it requires video-camera-audio systems, computers, servers, monitoring interfaces, sensors, and remote health devices [8].

Synchronous teleassessment is provided by healthcare providers using a video call session with the patient. At the same time, asynchronous is a type of teleassessment in which patients are monitored using digital medical devices, such as weight scales, blood pressure monitors, pulse oximeters, and blood glucose meters (see Fig. 5.2).

The potential of teleassessment methods in cardiopulmonary monitoring to improve the diagnosis and treatment of cardiovascular and respiratory diseases has attracted much attention. Remote Electrocardiography (tele-ECG) monitoring has emerged as a valuable tool for continuous and long-term heart health monitoring [9]. Research findings indicate that tele-ECG monitoring systems, such as wearable ECG patches, can accurately identify undiagnosed atrial fibrillation (AF) [10]. Furthermore, it has been found that tele-ECG increases the possibility of silent AF detection in ischemic stroke patients, improving the diagnostic yield and cost-effectiveness burden [11]. Likewise, tele-ECG monitoring has advanced, enabling real-time patient monitoring. This is due to the development of wearable remote ECG monitoring systems, optimized design based on artificial intelligence (AI) and Internet of Things (IoT), and encryption approaches for ECG monitoring systems [12, 13]. Smartphone-based ECG monitoring tools, such as the AliveCorTM heart monitor, have also shown sensitive and accurate single-lead ECG diagnosis of AF [14].

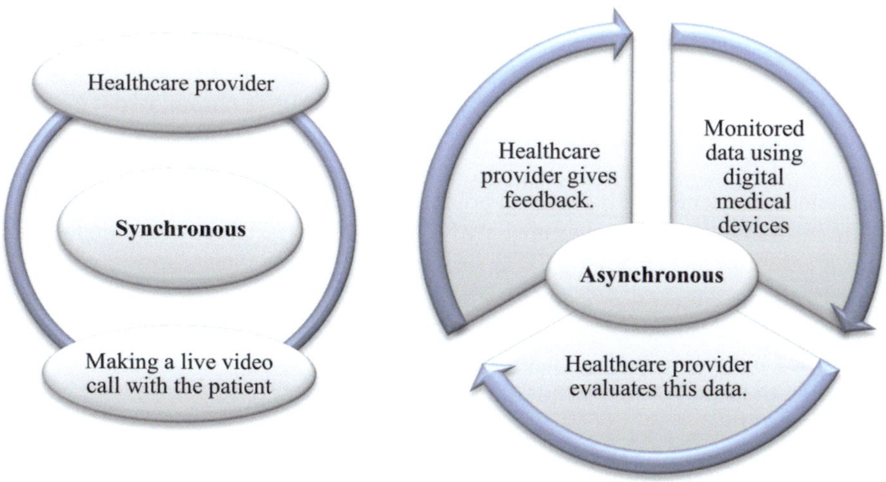

Fig. 5.2 Synchronous and asynchronous teleassessment

Additionally, reports of the effective detection of unknown paroxysmal atrial fibrillation have been made using wearables for heart rate and activity tracking, such as the Apple Watch. This shows the promise of consumer-grade wearables for remote cardiac monitoring [15]. Similarly, IoT-based systems for inductive sensor-based cardiac activity monitoring have been developed, which enable continuous ECG signal monitoring through electrodes attached to the skin [16]. Therefore, tele-ECG monitoring has shown great promise in detecting cardiac arrhythmias, improving clinical outcomes, and using fewer healthcare resources [17].

The ability of remote lung function testing, oxygen saturation monitoring, and wearable devices for activity tracking has attracted much attention, particularly considering the COVID-19 pandemic and chronic respiratory diseases. A cloud platform for remote pulmonary function testing with a smartphone microphone was introduced by Chung et al. [18], highlighting the possibility of remote pulmonary function monitoring. In addition, Fekr et al. [19] presented a medical cloud-based platform that measures respiration rate and classifies breath disorders hierarchically. This highlights the possibility of remote respiratory condition diagnosis and monitoring [19]. Soleimani et al. [20] showed the promise of depth-based lung function assessment and provided perspectives on technological developments that make remote lung function testing possible [20]. These findings support the increasing interest in lung function testing through remote technologies, especially in pandemics and respiratory diseases.

In conclusion, teleassessment technologies provide valuable instruments for continuously assessing cardiopulmonary health. These developments have the potential to completely change how cardiopulmonary diseases are diagnosed and treated, giving medical practitioners access to real-time data that will help them make better decisions and improve patient outcomes.

5.3 Integration of Artificial Intelligence (AI)

As technology evolves rapidly, every major innovation has the extraordinary potential to transform some aspect of society. In the age of ever-shrinking devices and smartphone apps, the constant flow of personalized information has become the standard of living. Similarly, adopting artificial intelligence (AI) in cardiopulmonary teleassessment has far-reaching potential [21–23].

In cardiology, machine learning (ML), a subset of artificial intelligence, has shown potential in analyzing cardiac imaging data [24]. AI has also been used for remote monitoring and waveform analysis in ECG, indicating its potential to improve cardiac care through teleassessment [25]. Moreover, AI has been used in emergency nursing to manage patients with chronic obstructive lung disease, demonstrating the value of this technology for remote patient management and pulmonary care [26].

The utilization of AI in remote cardiopulmonary assessments is consistent with the general trend of AI becoming increasingly used in medical applications, demonstrating remarkable outcomes and improvements in healthcare [27]. Furthermore,

AI's usefulness in remotely evaluating medical imaging data for cardiopulmonary assessments has been highlighted, showing its potential in remote interpretation and image understanding [28]. In summary, AI's proven efficacy in medical imaging analysis, remote patient monitoring, and diagnostics support its application in cardiopulmonary assessments remotely, emphasizing the technology's potential to improve the standard and efficacy of remote healthcare services.

5.4 Privacy, Data Security, Advantages, and Disadvantages

5.4.1 Privacy and Data Security

The widespread use of digital technologies and the Internet in healthcare services has brought cyber and technology-related data security and privacy exposures [29]. Privacy and data security are the whole of the efforts to protect the information as an asset without being exposed to any change, to protect it as a whole, to store it without being disclosed and shared, and to prevent unauthorized access. The primary purpose of privacy and data security is to ensure confidentiality, prevent unauthorized access, provide accessibility to authorized persons for the proper purpose and at the right time, and protect all these without being subject to any change [29]. Code/encryption/authentication processes should be used for privacy and data security. A summary of best practice recommendations is provided based on a new systematic review study shedding light on privacy and data security (see Table 5.1) [30].

Table 5.1 Privacy and data security recommendations for best practice of telehealth

Recommendations
• Determine steps to privacy and data security
• Input personal data only on safe websites indicated by a lock icon in the address bar
• All online meetings should need passwords, and while the patient is still in the waiting room, information should be verified
• Never schedule a telehealth consultation or provide personal information to an unidentified provider
• Keep your gadgets safe by using up-to-date antivirus software
• Do not access telehealth services using public Wi-Fi connections
• Do not use gadgets shared with people outside of the home or family when accessing telehealth services
• Optimize audio and video quality by collaborating with IT personnel to provide sufficient bandwidth
• Increase the Internet's speed by improving network use, service quality, and other strategies
• Provide resources and training to the patients with inadequate digital health proficiency

5.4.2 Teleassessment Advantages [31–34]

- Facilitates access to health services for patients living in rural areas far from the center. Thus, it is thought that inequality in the provision of health services can be reduced.
- Research has shown that telehealth applications can reduce time, health expenditures, and the economic burden of diseases.
- Enables faster and effortless sharing of medical information from patients to their relatives, caregivers, and healthcare professionals.
- Enables rapid evaluation of treatment efficacy and easier disease management.
- Even if there is no pandemic, it allows patients who cannot access healthcare for any reason to access health services.

5.4.3 Teleassessment Disadvantages [33, 35]

- Teleassessment services may reduce the reliability of assessment as they remove the objective influence of the health professional from many direct manual assessment and examination methods.
- It requires the patient to have adequate technological equipment and to know how to use it.
- Hardware and technological systems must be solved in case of possible problems that may negatively affect the healthcare process.
- Patient data privacy issues may arise (e.g., cyber data security).

5.5 Clinical Applications and Current Evidence

The COVID-19 pandemic and logistical and financial obstacles severely limited access to the healthcare system. Teleassessment methods are now employed instead of face-to-face assessment to help overcome the barriers to cardiopulmonary rehabilitation as information and communication technologies provide new alternatives in clinical evaluation [36]. In various cardiopulmonary diseases, such as chronic heart failure (CHF), cystic fibrosis (CF), chronic obstructive pulmonary disease (COPD), diabetes mellitus (DM), lung cancer, and COVID-19, outcome parameters, such as functional exercise capacity, frailty, muscle strength, and joint range of motion (ROM) were evaluated using technology-based teleassessment methods [37–46]. According to available data, several teleassessment methods for cardiopulmonary disease may provide a reliable, valid, and efficient substitute for a face-to-face assessment. A summary of the characteristics of validity and reliability studies of teleassessment in cardiopulmonary rehabilitation is shown in Table 5.2.

Table 5.2 Summary of characteristics of validity and/or reliability studies of teleassessment in cardiopulmonary rehabilitation

First author and year	Participants	Teleassessment environment and technology and outcome measure
Cox et al. (2013) [38]	Cystic fibrosis	Simulated telehealth environment/synchronous videoconference/submaximal exercise capacity (the 3-min step test)
Galiano-Castillo et al. (2014) [47]	Breast cancer survivors	Simulated telehealth environment/synchronous videoconference/arm measurements via a telehealth application
Hwang et al. (2016) [39]	Chronic heart failure	Simulated telehealth environment/synchronous videoconference/functional exercise capacity (6MWT, TUG, and grip strength)
Wood et al. (2017) [48]	Cystic fibrosis	Telehealth clinic/synchronous videoconference/health outcomes (Cystic Fibrosis Questionnaire)
Exum et al. (2020) [49]	COVID-19	Consultations performed remotely or outside/synchronous videoconference or telephone consultations
Mukaino et al. (2020) [41]	COVID-19	Isolated hospital room/synchronous videoconference/vital signs (pulse oximeter) and levels of functioning (Functional Independence Measure)
Wootton et al. (2020) [50]	COVID-19	Home setting/synchronous videoconference/5-repetitive STS and 1-min STS, and dyspnea, fatigue, and other symptoms via monitor
Zahiri et al. (2020) [45]	Chronic obstructive pulmonary disease	Clinic environment/based on a tablet with a camera module/physical frailty (sensorless frailty meter)
López-López et al. (2022) [40]	After COVID-19 in non-hospitalized patients	Synchronous videoconference/lower limb function (SPPB), upper limb function (maximal number of shoulder flexions), exercise capacity (30-s STS test), symptoms before-after test (dyspnea and fatigue 0–10)
Ozsoy et al. (2022) [42]	Chronic obstructive pulmonary disease	Home/synchronized videoconference and asynchronized/functionality and lower limb capacity ((TUG), and 5-repetitive STS test), perception of dyspnea and fatigue severity (using the modified Borg scale), cardiorespiratory responses (SpO_2 and heart rate)
Heredia-Ciuró et al. (2022) [43]	Lung cancer survivors	Home/synchronous videoconference/upper limb function (Shirt Task) and musculoskeletal disturbances (active ROM and trigger points)
Aktan et al. (2023) [37]	Diabetes mellitus type 2	Synchronous videoconference/functional exercise capacity (30-s STS), perception of dyspnea and fatigue severity (modified Borg scale), cardiorespiratory responses (SpO_2, blood pressure, and heart rate)

(continued)

Table 5.2 (continued)

First author and year	Participants	Teleassessment environment and technology and outcome measure
Pepera et al. (2023) [44]	Diabetes mellitus type 2	Outside each patient's home/synchronous videoconference/functional capacity (6MWT) and cardiorespiratory responses (blood pressure, heart rate, and SpO_2 using an electronic sphygmomanometer)
Yilmaz Gokmen et al. (2023) [46]	Hospitalized/ non-hospitalized COVID-19 survivors	Synchronous videoconference/functional capacity (30-second STS) and general clinical condition (C19-YRS Tool)

6MWT 6-minute walk test, *TUG* timed up-and-go tests, *STS* sit-to-stand tests, *SPPB* short physical performance battery, *SpO_2* peripheral oxygen saturation, *C19-YRS* the COVID-19 Yorkshire rehabilitation screening tool

5.5.1 Functional Exercise Capacity and Cardiorespiratory Responses

Teleassessment methods are widely used to measure functional exercise capacity in cardiopulmonary diseases to overcome obstacles preventing patients from accessing physiotherapy practices. Teleassessments and traditional face-to-face assessments have been compared using the 6-minute walk test (6MWT), timed up-and-go tests (TUG), and grip strength tests in patients with CHF [39]. Evaluation of functional exercise capacity by teleassessment methods in patients with CHF is considered valid and reliable. Similarly, 6MWT performed outdoors via teleassessment is a reliable and valid tool for evaluating functional exercise capacity in patients with DM type 2.

One of the most popular and straightforward techniques for evaluating functional exercise capacity in patients with CF is the 3-minute step test, which requires little space and equipment [51]. In addition, the validity and reliability of teleassessment via remote video monitoring of the 3-minute step test were also examined by comparing it with face-to-face assessment in patients with CF. It has been stated that utilizing the 3-minute step test through video-based teleassessment is accurate and practicable for functional exercise capacity assessment in patients with CF [38]. Cardiopulmonary diseases, including COPD and DM, are commonly assessed for lower extremity physical performance and functional exercise capacity using the 30-second sit-to-stand (STS), 5-repetitive STS, and TUG tests [37, 42, 46]. Özsoy et al. [42] reported TUG and 5-repetitive STS tests in patients with COPD as reproducible teleassessment measurements with excellent intra- and inter-rater reliability. Similarly, Aktan et al. [37] showed a high level of inter-rater reliability between the teleassessment of the 30-second STS test and face-to-face assessment methods in patients with DM type 2. These results suggest that the 30-second STS test teleassessment for DM type 2 patients and the TUG and 5-repetitive STS test teleassessment for COPD patients are valid and valuable tools for assessing functional exercise capacity. Furthermore, the 30-second STS test teleassessment approach was used in a few research to assess functional exercise ability in hospitalized/

non-hospitalized COVID-19 patients. It seems that COVID-19 patients can benefit from the reliable usage of 30-second STS real-time teleassessment [40, 46].

Cardiorespiratory responses, including heart rate, blood pressure, peripheral oxygen saturation (SpO_2), perceived dyspnea, and fatigue severity, are typically examined in functional exercise capacity tests, whether conducted through teleassessment or traditional face-to-face assessment. Pulse oximeters connected to a tablet computer via Bluetooth are often used to measure cardiorespiratory responses in teleassessment. Cardiorespiratory responses and changes measured by teleassessment and center-based assessments of functional exercise capacity generally reveal similar results [37, 38]. However, the location of the teleassessment is a crucial detail to remember in this case. By enhancing the patient's sense of trust, teleassessments by physiotherapists in different rooms within the same building may lead to better results. Additionally, there can be a difference in the cardiorespiratory responses, such as SpO_2 and dyspnea, between the two approaches if face-to-face assessment is conducted indoors/clinic and teleassessment is conducted outdoors [44]. Therefore, a key element in ensuring the validity and usefulness of the tests is optimizing the setting for teleassessment techniques in cardiopulmonary physiotherapy.

5.5.2 Lower-Upper Limb Function and Range of Motion

Teleassessment methods for the musculoskeletal system, such as ROM, muscular strength, and function of the lower and upper extremities, have been applied in several cardiopulmonary disease populations [39, 40, 42–44]. Lower extremity function was assessed using the Short Physical Performance Battery (SPPB) in COVID-19 patients. The teleassessment and face-to-face assessment of the SPPB has been shown to have excellent inter-rater reliability [40]. Furthermore, to assess upper limb function in lung cancer survivors, the Shirt Task, active ROM with photogrammetry, and trigger points with self-explanation, both face-to-face and teleassessment methods were used [43]. It demonstrated the inter-rater solid reliability of upper extremity teleassessment methods used by physical therapists to evaluate musculoskeletal problems and upper extremity function in lung cancer survivors. Similarly, upper extremity function was assessed with a free weight (1 kg) in the hands and the maximum number of shoulder flexions in 1 min with the teleassessment method in COVID-19 patients [40]. Thus, upper and lower extremity functions and related parameters in different cardiopulmonary diseases can be evaluated by teleassessment methods.

5.5.3 Questionnaires (Fatigue, Dyspnea, Quality of Life, and Functional Level)

In assessing cardiopulmonary diseases, questionnaires and scales commonly measure characteristics such as fatigue, dyspnea, functional level, and overall or disease-specific health-related quality of life (HRQoL) [37, 40–42, 46, 48]. The modified Borg Scale yielded similar results when face-to-face and teleassessment approaches were used to evaluate the perceived severity of dyspnea and fatigue in cardiopulmonary diseases. Thus, in teleassessment, the modified Borg scale can be utilized with confidence [37]. Furthermore, scales directly measured by the teleassessment approach have also been created. For instance, a multidisciplinary team working in post-COVID-19 rehabilitation services developed the COVID-19 Yorkshire Rehabilitation Screening (C19-YRS) Tool, a telephone assessment/screening tool made up of questions on the general clinical status of COVID-19 survivors [52]. Furthermore, the Functional Independence Scale (FIM) was used teleassessment to examine the functional levels of COVID-19 patients [41]. Patients with CF had their disease-specific HRQoL measured via teleassessment using the Cystic Fibrosis Questionnaire (CFQ) [48]. Accordingly, research on several cardiopulmonary diseases suggests that teleassessment methods could provide a safe and reliable substitute for examination in centers.

5.6 Patient Engagement and Satisfaction

Teleassessment methods can improve access and enable accessible communication with healthcare professionals, reducing travel time, cost, and wait times for healthcare. Along with all of these advantages, it's critical to emphasize that, as far as patient safety is concerned, no adverse events related to teleassessments have been documented in any of the studies done [36]. In the cardiopulmonary field, patient satisfaction reports using teleassessment techniques have been made for COVID-19, CF, and CHF patients. Studies using satisfaction surveys, such as the Telemedicine Satisfaction Questionnaire and the System Usability Scale, to assess participant satisfaction with teleassessments have found that overall satisfaction was high [38, 39, 41, 53]. Furthermore, it is noteworthy that there is no difference in satisfaction levels between face-to-face assessment, teleassessment, and combined service types when compared; in fact, the teleassessment method exhibits a higher level of satisfaction, particularly regarding convenience in scheduling appointments [53].

5.7 Future Directions and Innovations

5.7.1 Emerging Technologies in Cardiopulmonary Teleassessment

With the increasing accessibility of digital health tools such as wearable technologies and smartphone applications used in medical practices, digital health applications are gaining more attention in preventing and managing cardiovascular diseases, frailty, and 6MWT [54, 55]. The risk of frailty and cardiovascular disease is being identified and prevented with the increased use of teleassessment techniques [55]. Furthermore, the remote screening of physical frailty is one of the emerging technologies in cardiopulmonary teleassessment procedures [45]. A deep learning-based image processing-based sensorless frailty meter (FM) was created. It is simple to integrate into mobile health and enables remote evaluation of physical frailty. Furthermore, the 6MWT application can also be used remotely at home to monitor heart patients' functional exercise capacities [54]. Teleassessment methods and developing technologies may be more beneficial for cardiopulmonary patients whose access is limited due to distance or clinical characteristics.

5.7.2 Potential Impact of Virtual Reality and Augmented Reality in Telemedicine

Virtual reality (VR)-based diagnostics and treatments are becoming more and more common due to growing needs and technological advances, particularly in cardiac disease [56]. Specifically, wearable, unconnected holographic computers that provide video, audio, and mixed reality (MR) composites for two-way communication with numerous remote users have been deployed [57]. This technology has been applied in preoperative planning, surgical training, anatomical teaching, and 3D telemedicine support, among other clinical and educational contexts. Data on teleassessment methods with the help of VR in cardiopulmonary physiotherapy are currently lacking. But as long as technology keeps improving, the use of VR, MR, and artificial intelligence-supported cardiopulmonary teleassessment methods will soon take their place in the literature and clinical practice.

5.8 Conclusion

5.8.1 Summarizing the Improvements in Cardiopulmonary Teleassessment

Various types of physiotherapy measurement are performed using teleassessment methods in cardiopulmonary diseases, and the most often used teleassessment methods include 5-repetition STS, 30-second STS, TUG, 6MWT, ROM, and disease-specific HRQoL scales. Functional exercise capacity, cardiorespiratory responses, physical function, muscle strength, frailty, ROM, and HRQoL questionnaires seem valid and reliable in cardiopulmonary diseases. It is also seen that patients are satisfied with teleassessment methods in the field of cardiac rehabilitation. However, most studies on teleassessment in cardiopulmonary physiotherapy have focused on specific disease groups such as COVID-19, DM, CF, and CHF with small sample sizes. Therefore, since the acceptability of physiotherapy assessments among teleassessment methods varies with each cardiopulmonary disease, it would be incorrect to generalize each teleassessment method to different cardiopulmonary disease groups. In light of the global trend towards teleassessment, further extensive research with bigger sample sizes is required in cardiopulmonary physiotherapy.

Table 5.3 Implications for future healthcare practices

A protocol for the management of potential adverse events should be devised, and patients should be carefully chosen, to prevent significant adverse events during teleassessment
Surveys should be used to inquire about patients' experiences and satisfaction with teleassessment methods and any required adjustments should be made in response to the findings
To lessen patient demand and audio feedback, more sophisticated technological resources like Bluetooth and wireless headsets should be provided during teleassessments
New advances in technology mean that more should be made use of infrastructure and hardware support, such as improved videoconferencing software, artificial intelligence capabilities, and faster Internet connection
Technology should be used in the reporting section as well as in the measurement of cardiorespiratory responses. During teleassessments, the introduction of valid and trustworthy wearable sensors-like sports or smartwatches may help to provide a more objective evaluation of cardiorespiratory reactions
Mobile data support is required for outdoor teleassessment, and technical issues should be avoided. By making sure the family member or medical professional participates in the evaluations, potential technical issues can be avoided. On the other hand, we think that in the future, apps based on artificial intelligence will help this problem
If equipment is needed for teleassessments, a uniform measuring technique or protocol should be developed utilizing the same kind of remote monitoring and assessment apparatus
Future studies should look into the viability of remote assessments in various indoor and outdoor settings, especially as it relates to how various external factors like weather and air pollution may affect outdoor tests

5.8.2 Implications for Future Healthcare Practices

Implications for future healthcare practices are summarized in Table 5.3.

Conflicts of Interest The authors have no conflicts of interest to declare that are relevant to the content of this chapter. Also, all figures and tables used are original and not obtained from anywhere else.

References

1. Ceravolo MG, de Sire A, Andrenelli E, Negrini F, Negrini S. Systematic rapid "living" review on rehabilitation needs due to COVID-19: update to March 31st, 2020. Eur J Phys Rehabil Med. 2020;56(3):347–53.
2. Galea MD. Telemedicine in rehabilitation. Phys Med Rehabil Clin N Am. 2019;30(2):473–83.
3. Scherrenberg M, Wilhelm M, Hansen D, Völler H, Cornelissen V, Frederix I, et al. The future is now: a call for action for cardiac telerehabilitation in the COVID-19 pandemic from the secondary prevention and rehabilitation section of the European Association of Preventive Cardiology. Eur J Prev Cardiol. 2021;28(5):524–40.
4. Carda S, Invernizzi M, Bavikatte G, Bensmaïl D, Bianchi F, Deltombe T, et al. The role of physical and rehabilitation medicine in the COVID-19 pandemic: the clinician's view. Ann Phys Rehabil Med. 2020;63(6):554–6.
5. Krach SK, Paskiewicz TL, Monk MM. Testing our children when the world shuts down: analyzing recommendations for adapted tele-assessment during COVID-19. J Psychoeduc Assess. 2020;38(8):923–41.

6. Yıldırım Şahan T. Telerehabilitasyon. In: Demirgüç A, editor. Sağlıkta ve Hastalıkta Egzersiz 1 Baskı. Ankara: Türkiye Klinikleri; 2021. p. 76–81.
7. Purssell E, Gould D, Chudleigh J. Impact of isolation on hospitalised patients who are infectious: systematic review with meta-analysis. BMJ Open. 2020;10(2):e030371.
8. Prvu Bettger J, Resnik LJ. Telerehabilitation in the age of COVID-19: an opportunity for learning health system research. Phys Ther. 2020;100(11):1913–6.
9. Rateb AM. A fast compressed sensing decoding technique for remote ECG monitoring systems. IEEE Access. 2020;8:197124–33.
10. Steinhubl SR, Waalen J, Edwards AM, Ariniello LM, Mehta RR, Ebner GS, et al. Effect of a home-based wearable continuous ECG monitoring patch on detection of undiagnosed atrial fibrillation: the mSToPS randomized clinical trial. JAMA. 2018;320(2):146–55.
11. Grond M, Jauss M, Hamann G, Stark E, Veltkamp R, Nabavi D, et al. Improved detection of silent atrial fibrillation using 72-hour Holter ECG in patients with ischemic stroke. Stroke. 2013;44(12):3357–64.
12. Yin M, Tang R, Liu M, Han K, Lv X, Huang M, et al. Influence of optimization design based on artificial intelligence and internet of things on the electrocardiogram monitoring system. J Healthc Eng. 2020;2020:8840910.
13. Zheng L, Wang Z, Tian S. Comparative study on electrocardiogram encryption using elliptic curves cryptography and data encryption standard for applications in Internet of medical things. Concurr Comput Pract Exp. 2022;34(9):e5776.
14. Tu HT, Chen Z, Swift C, Churilov L, Guo R, Liu X, et al. Smartphone electrographic monitoring for atrial fibrillation in acute ischemic stroke and transient ischemic attack. Int J Stroke. 2017;12(7):786–9.
15. Hirota K, Hirai M. Apple watch for pulse rate assessment detects unidentified paroxysmal atrial fibrillation. Reports. 2022;5(4):40.
16. Brezulianu A, Geman O, Zbancioc MD, Hagan M, Aghion C, Hemanth DJ, et al. IoT based heart activity monitoring using inductive sensors. Sensors. 2019;19(15):3284.
17. Chiu CSL, Timmermans I, Versteeg H, Zitron E, Mabo P, Pedersen SS, et al. Effect of remote monitoring on clinical outcomes in European heart failure patients with an implantable cardioverter-defibrillator: secondary results of the REMOTE-CIED randomized trial. EP Europace. 2021;24(2):256–67.
18. Chung H, Jeong C, Luhach AK, Nam Y, Lee J. Remote pulmonary function test monitoring in cloud platform via smartphone built-in microphone. Evol Bioinforma. 2019;15:1176934319888904.
19. Fekr AR, Janidarmian M, Radecka K, Zilic Z. A medical cloud-based platform for respiration rate measurement and hierarchical classification of breath disorders. Sensors. 2014;14(6):11204–24.
20. Soleimani V, Mirmehdi M, Damen D, Dodd J, Hannuna S, Sharp C, et al. Remote, depth-based lung function assessment. IEEE Trans Biomed Eng. 2017;64(8):1943–58.
21. Seetharam K, Brito D, Farjo PD, Sengupta PP. The role of artificial intelligence in cardiovascular imaging: state of the art review. Front Cardiovasc Med. 2020;7:618849.
22. Johnson KW, Torres Soto J, Glicksberg BS, Shameer K, Miotto R, Ali M, et al. Artificial intelligence in cardiology. J Am Coll Cardiol. 2018;71(23):2668–79.
23. Seetharam K, Kagiyama N, Sengupta PP. Application of mobile health, telemedicine and artificial intelligence to echocardiography. Echo Res Pract. 2019;6(2):R41–52.
24. Seetharam K, Shrestha S, Sengupta PP. Artificial intelligence in cardiac imaging. US Cardiol Rev. 2019;13(2):110–6.
25. Nedadur R, Wang B, Yanagawa B. The cardiac surgeon's guide to artificial intelligence. Curr Opin Cardiol. 2021;36(5):637–43.
26. Hong L, Cheng X, Zheng D. Application of artificial intelligence in emergency nursing of patients with chronic obstructive pulmonary disease. Contrast Media Mol Imaging. 2021;2021:6423398.
27. Jiao L, Huang Z, Liu X, Yang Y, Ma M, Zhao J, et al. Brain-inspired remote sensing interpretation: a comprehensive survey. IEEE J Sel Top Appl Earth Obs Remote Sens. 2023;16:2992–3033.

28. Jia S-C, Wang T. Research on shadow detection method of infrared remote sensing image based on artificial intelligence. In: Zhang Y-D, Wang S-H, Liu S, editors. Multimedia technology and enhanced learning. Cham: Springer International Publishing; 2020. p. 426–36.
29. Britton KE, Britton-Colonnese JD. Privacy and security issues surrounding the protection of data generated by continuous glucose monitors. J Diabetes Sci Technol. 2017;11(2):216–9.
30. Houser SH, Flite CA, Foster SL. Privacy and security risk factors related to telehealth services—a systematic review. Perspect Health Inf Manag. 2023;20(1):1f.
31. Hailey D, Roine R, Ohinmaa A, Dennett L. Evidence of benefit from telerehabilitation in routine care: a systematic review. J Telemed Telecare. 2011;17(6):281–7.
32. Rogante M, Grigioni M, Cordella D, Giacomozzi C. Ten years of telerehabilitation: a literature overview of technologies and clinical applications. NeuroRehabilitation. 2010;27(4):287–304.
33. Russell TG. Telerehabilitation: a coming of age. Aust J Physiother. 2009;55(1):5–6.
34. Burns RB, Crislip D, Daviou P, Temkin A, Vesmarovich S, Anshutz J, et al. Using telerehabilitation to support assistive technology. Assist Technol. 1998;10(2):126–33.
35. Richmond T, Peterson C, Cason J, Billings M, Terrell EA, Lee ACW, et al. American Telemedicine Association's principles for delivering telerehabilitation services. Int J Telerehabil. 2017;9(2):63–8.
36. Zischke C, Simas V, Hing W, Milne N, Spittle A, Pope R. The utility of physiotherapy assessments delivered by telehealth: a systematic review. J Glob Health. 2021;11:04072.
37. Aktan R, Yılmaz H, Demir İ, Özalevli S. Agreement between tele-assessment and face-to-face assessment of 30-s sit-to-stand test in patients with type 2 diabetes mellitus. Ir J Med Sci. 2023;192(5):2173–8.
38. Cox NS, Alison JA, Button BM, Wilson JW, Holland AE. Assessing exercise capacity using telehealth: a feasibility study in adults with cystic fibrosis. Respir Care. 2013;58(2):286–90.
39. Hwang R, Mandrusiak A, Morris NR, Peters R, Korczyk D, Russell T. Assessing functional exercise capacity using telehealth: is it valid and reliable in patients with chronic heart failure? J Telemed Telecare. 2017;23(2):225–32.
40. López-López L, Beas-Cobo F, Ortiz-Rubio A, Martín-Núñez J, Calvache-Mateo A, Heredia-Ciuró A, et al. Agreement between face-to-face and tele-assessment of physical function measurement after COVID-19 in non-hospitalized patients. Eur J Phys Rehabil Med. 2022;58(5):784–5.
41. Mukaino M, Tatemoto T, Kumazawa N, Tanabe S, Katoh M, Saitoh E, et al. An affordable, user-friendly telerehabilitation system assembled using existing technologies for individuals isolated with COVID-19: development and feasibility study. JMIR Rehabil Assist Technol. 2020;7(2):e24960.
42. Ozsoy I, Kodak MI, Kararti C, Ozsoy G, Erturk A, Kahraman T. Intra- and inter-rater reproducibility of the face-to-face and tele-assessment of Timed-Up and Go and 5-Times Sit-to-Stand tests in patients with chronic obstructive pulmonary disease. COPD. 2022;19(1):125–32.
43. Heredia-Ciuró A, Lazo-Prados A, Blasco-Valls P, Calvache-Mateo A, Lopez-Lopez L, Martin-Nuñez J, et al. Agreement between face-to-face and tele-assessment of upper limb disability in lung cancer survivors during COVID-19 era. J Telemed Telecare. 2024;30(4):668–74. https://doi.org/10.1177/1357633X221079543.
44. Pepera G, Karanasiou E, Blioumpa C, Antoniou V, Kalatzis K, Lanaras L, et al. Tele-assessment of functional capacity through the Six-Minute Walk Test in patients with diabetes mellitus type 2: validity and reliability of repeated measurements. Sensors (Basel). 2023;23(3):1354.
45. Zahiri M, Wang C, Gardea M, Nguyen H, Shahbazi M, Sharafkhaneh A, et al. Remote physical frailty monitoring-the application of deep learning-based image processing in tele-health. IEEE Access. 2020;8:219391–9.
46. Yilmaz Gokmen G, Durmaz D, Demir C, Yilmaz FN. Determining post-COVID-19 symptoms and rehabilitation needs in hospitalized and nonhospitalized COVID-19 survivors with tele-assessment methods. Telemed J E Health. 2023;29(9):1312–23.
47. Galiano-Castillo N, Ariza-García A, Cantarero-Villanueva I, Fernández-Lao C, Sánchez-Salado C, Arroyo-Morales M. Agreement between telerehabilitation involving caregivers

and face-to-face clinical assessment of lymphedema in breast cancer survivors. Support Care Cancer. 2014;22(1):253–8.
48. Wood J, Mulrennan S, Hill K, Cecins N, Morey S, Jenkins S. Telehealth clinics increase access to care for adults with cystic fibrosis living in rural and remote Western Australia. J Telemed Telecare. 2017;23(7):673–9.
49. Exum E, Hull BL, Lee ACW, Gumieny A, Villarreal C, Longnecker D. Applying telehealth technologies and strategies to provide acute care consultation and treatment of patients with confirmed or possible COVID-19. J Acute Care Phys Ther. 2020;11(3) https://doi.org/10.1097/JAT.0000000000000143.
50. Wootton SL, King M, Alison JA, Mahadev S, Chan ASL. COVID-19 rehabilitation delivered via a telehealth pulmonary rehabilitation model: a case series. Respirol Case Rep. 2020;8(8):e00669.
51. Balfour-Lynn IM, Prasad SA, Laverty A, Whitehead BF, Dinwiddie R. A step in the right direction: assessing exercise tolerance in cystic fibrosis. Pediatr Pulmonol. 1998;25(4):278–84.
52. Sivan M, Halpin S, Gee J. Assessing long-term rehabilitation needs in COVID-19 survivors using a telephone screening tool (C19-YRS tool). Adv Clin Neurosci Rehabil. 2020;19(4):14–7.
53. Eannucci EF, Hazel K, Grundstein MJ, Nguyen JT, Gallegro J. Patient satisfaction for telehealth physical therapy services was comparable to that of in-person services during the COVID-19 pandemic. HSS J. 2020;16(Suppl 1):10–6.
54. Scherrenberg M, Bonneux C, Yousif Mahmood D, Hansen D, Dendale P, Coninx K. A Mobile application to perform the Six-Minute Walk Test (6MWT) at home: a random walk in the park is as accurate as a standardized 6MWT. Sensors (Basel). 2022;22(11):4277.
55. Guasti L, Dilaveris P, Mamas MA, Richter D, Christodorescu R, Lumens J, et al. Digital health in older adults for the prevention and management of cardiovascular diseases and frailty. A clinical consensus statement from the ESC Council for Cardiology Practice/Taskforce on Geriatric Cardiology, the ESC Digital Health Committee and the ESC Working Group on e-Cardiology. ESC Heart Fail. 2022;9(5):2808–22.
56. Cen J, Liufu R, Wen S, Qiu H, Liu X, Chen X, et al. Three-dimensional printing, virtual reality and mixed reality for pulmonary atresia: early surgical outcomes evaluation. Heart Lung Circ. 2021;30(2):296–302.
57. Martin G, Koizia L, Kooner A, Cafferkey J, Ross C, Purkayastha S, et al. Use of the HoloLens2 mixed reality headset for protecting health care workers during the COVID-19 pandemic: prospective, observational evaluation. J Med Internet Res. 2020;22(8):e21486.

Telerehabilitation Methods in Cardiopulmonary Rehabilitation

6

Selver Nalbant, Emine Korkmaz, and Baki Umut Tuğay

6.1 Pulmonary Rehabilitation

6.1.1 Pulmonary Diseases and Pulmonary Rehabilitation

Chronic respiratory diseases represent a significant health issue globally, contributing to 7% of the global disease burden. Among these diseases, chronic obstructive pulmonary disease (COPD), interstitial lung diseases (ILDs), bronchiectasis, and chronic asthma are prominent. Pulmonary rehabilitation provided for managing these conditions plays a crucial role in enhancing patients' quality of life and improving health outcomes [1].

Pulmonary rehabilitation programs include various components such as aerobic exercise, strength training, flexibility exercises, inspiratory muscle training, and respiratory education. These programs are tailored by combining personalized aerobic exercise, strength training in the upper and lower extremities, flexibility exercises for improving thoracic mobility and posture, and respiratory education to reduce dyspnea and dynamic hyperinflation. These components are integrated with disease-specific education and self-management skills to form comprehensive rehabilitation programs [2–5]. Participation and continuity in exercises and educational

S. Nalbant
Department of Physiotherapy and Rehabilitation, Bucak School of Health, Burdur Mehmet Akif Ersoy University, Burdur, Turkey

E. Korkmaz
Department of Physical Therapy and Rehabilitation, Muğla Training and Research Hospital, Muğla, Turkey

B. U. Tuğay (✉)
Department of Physiotherapy and Rehabilitation, Faculty of Health Sciences, Muğla Sıtkı Koçman University, Muğla, Turkey
e-mail: umutt@mu.edu.tr

F. Özden et al. (eds.), *Telerehabilitation*, TELe-Health,
https://doi.org/10.1007/978-3-031-69080-8_6

sessions are crucial for achieving optimal gains throughout the rehabilitation program. Despite pulmonary rehabilitation's well-known benefits and outcomes, research and clinical practices demonstrate low participant engagement, inadequate continuity, and high dropout rates [6, 7].

6.1.2 Telerehabilitation in Pulmonary Rehabilitation

The development and increased availability of communication technologies have led to the emergence of technology-based enhanced healthcare delivery methods, whether in hospital settings, home environments, or post-discharge scenarios [8]. Telehealth interventions involve the provision of healthcare services through the use of telecommunication or virtual technology tools [9]. The World Health Organization defines telehealth and applications as providing remote healthcare services using information and communication technologies by patients and healthcare providers [9]. These healthcare methods, or telemedicine or telehealth systems, have been adapted to rehabilitation fields [8]. Telerehabilitation is a domain aimed at remotely delivering clinical rehabilitation services, utilizing information and communication technologies for this purpose [10]. The utilization of telerehabilitation systems varies among countries, societies, and institutions [8].

Telerehabilitation is utilized in physical therapy for orthopedic, neurological, cardiac, and pulmonary system problems, with reports indicating better outcomes than traditional rehabilitation programs or no rehabilitation at all [11]. Various health technologies such as tele-monitoring, teleconsultation, tele-education, and telehealth are employed in treating pulmonary diseases, including pulmonary rehabilitation [12]. These methods utilize telecommunication technologies to deliver various components and aspects of pulmonary rehabilitation programs to patients in their homes or other suitable locations. Pulmonary telerehabilitation appears to yield outcomes similar to traditional center-based pulmonary rehabilitation. Considering that chronic respiratory diseases rank as the third leading cause of death globally, telerehabilitation is thought to be a significant tool in managing these conditions [12, 13]. Different program models include center-based telerehabilitation, which involves delivering exercise training and education programs in remote centers or centers with limited access to specialized centers; home-based rehabilitation, providing supervised rehabilitation in patients' home environments; and internet-based telerehabilitation models, which implement rehabilitation programs on different platforms such as mobile phones and internet applications [2, 14].

In numerous studies aiming to support pulmonary rehabilitation, the effectiveness and safety of telerehabilitation methods have been evaluated using various types of technology. These assessments compared telerehabilitation with center-based (outpatient) pulmonary rehabilitation, inpatient pulmonary rehabilitation, and control groups without rehabilitation. Telerehabilitation has been reported to have no adverse effects compared to face-to-face or no rehabilitation. However, similar outcomes have been observed when telerehabilitation applications are compared with other rehabilitation methods [13]. Numerous studies focusing on chronic obstructive pulmonary disease (COPD) have been conducted to determine the effectiveness of telerehabilitation in pulmonary rehabilitation. It has been confirmed that telerehabilitation methods yield improvements compared to traditional rehabilitation in symptoms and impairments associated with COPD and other pulmonary diseases, such as dyspnea, decreased functional capacity, and reduced quality of life. Regarding factors such as exercise capacity, maximal oxygen uptake, and quality of life, telerehabilitation appears comparable to other rehabilitation models in individuals with cardiopulmonary diseases. However, it is acknowledged that the current literature is limited regarding the long-term effects of telerehabilitation practices [14–16].

6.1.3 Telerehabilitation Methods in Pulmonary Rehabilitation

In pulmonary diseases, telerehabilitation applications encompass various methods, including mobile health technologies (mHealth), virtual exercise sessions, videoconferencing platforms, wearable devices, sensors, tele-education systems incorporating instructional videos and interactive modules, teleconsultations, and virtual examinations. These methods enhance access to rehabilitation, improve participation and adherence, optimize clinical outcomes, and enhance health and well-being. Mobile health technologies are increasingly becoming prevalent as critical facilitators in promoting behavioral change and serving as essential drivers in improving health outcomes. The World Health Organization defines mHealth as encompassing all monitoring devices, digital assistants, and wired and wireless devices, ranging from using mobile phones for voice and text messaging services to using third- and fourth-generation mobile telecommunication systems. These technologies are utilized in medical and public health applications, varying across different categories such as call centers, emergency management, mobile appointment and reminder systems, treatment adherence, patient monitoring systems, mobile health surveys, and decision support systems, depending on the level of development of countries and communities [17, 18].

Another device used in telerehabilitation is remote monitoring. Smartphone applications, wearable health technologies (such as smartwatches and skin patches), accelerometers, and standard pedometers are commonly used for measuring various health parameters, especially those related to physiological functioning (such as pulse, body temperature, heart rhythm, blood pressure, sleep quality, and stress level). Additionally, mHealth technologies include health coach telecommunication and health and wellness websites [19–22].

The use of smartphone applications for exercise education also facilitates exercise program planning. Technologies such as digital exercise diary, scheduled virtual group exercise sessions, exercise videos, and applications with virtual peer support and friend group functions for exercise education promote participation motivation, daily physical activity, and exercise education motivation in individuals with pulmonary diseases through peer and friend support [23]. Digital exercise logs and scheduled virtual group exercise sessions help avoid postponing exercise education. Furthermore, mHealth interventions based on behavior change theories (such as WeChat groups and web-based health education lectures) improve self-care management behaviors, thus enhancing the prevention and control of the pulmonary disease [24].

6.1.4 Advantages of Telerehabilitation in Pulmonary Rehabilitation

Improving access to pulmonary rehabilitation for patients and clients through different service models can enhance health outcomes and reduce hospitalization and healthcare utilization rates for individuals with chronic respiratory diseases [13]. Significant patient-centered challenges that hinder participation and completion of pulmonary rehabilitation often relate to travel and transportation to the rehabilitation center [25, 26]. Particularly in rural areas, access to pulmonary rehabilitation remains limited due to service shortages and a scarcity of trained healthcare professionals [27]. Factors associated with participation in pulmonary rehabilitation programs include travel expenses and transportation, perceived benefits, smoking habits, depression, disruption of regular routines, and program schedule [25, 26].

Studies support that telerehabilitation applications increase participation in pulmonary rehabilitation by alleviating the burden of travel, providing program flexibility, and addressing geographical disparities [28]. Pulmonary telerehabilitation emerges as a safe, cost-effective, and convenient alternative to traditional rehabilitation programs, particularly regarding logistics and finances [29]. Additionally, providing exercise education support solely through tablet computers increases participant completion rates and program participation compared to conventional rehabilitation programs [30]. Moreover, patient satisfaction is higher with telerehabilitation programs compared to traditional ones. It has been reported that satisfaction with future telerehabilitation programs is also supported [31]. Patient satisfaction is associated with disease-related programs and access to efficient and affordable healthcare services [32].

6.1.5 Disadvantages of Telerehabilitation in Pulmonary Rehabilitation

When pulmonary rehabilitation programs are delivered as telerehabilitation applications, they must maintain key treatment components such as exercise education, training, and behavior change programs. However, challenges are encountered, particularly in standardizing equipment and intervention designs. Therefore, international organizations related to the fields, such as the European Respiratory Society (ERS) and the American Thoracic Society (ATS), have reported the need for collaborative efforts among scientific and national organizations to standardize and enhance pulmonary telerehabilitation programs [33].

Remote rehabilitation methods present challenges, such as providing the initial assessment of the patient and delivering critical components of exercise prescription remotely [34]. While co-treatment with the traditional program can be achieved, palpation and manipulation are limited [8]. Additionally, limitations arise from Internet access, the usability of telesystems for all, and patient willingness [8, 29].

Telerehabilitation applications, telemedicine, and telehealth systems are commonly utilized in advanced societies [8, 35]. Similar to traditional rehabilitation programs, collaboration with technology experts is required to enable the remote provision of systems, such as respiratory monitors, pulse oximeters, sensors, and physiological variable monitors, with costs. The uncertainty regarding the cost-effectiveness of the systems and the expensiveness of some telemedicine system models also creates limitations in usage [8, 33].

Participants face challenges in learning and using technology. Patients with poorer health status and limited digital technology experience need help participating in and maintaining exercise programs. Therefore, there is a need to improve the simplicity and usability of all technology-based applications and devices [36–38]. Online security concerns pose another limitation to participation in programs. Mainly, there needs to be more regulation regarding commercially available mHealth applications [18].

6.1.6 Pulmonary Telerehabilitation Methods in a COVID and Post-COVID-19

The COVID-19 pandemic has highlighted both pulmonary growth and the expansion of telerehabilitation during crises of the period [39]. National and international guidelines have recommended the cessation of traditional pulmonary rehabilitation programs during and after the COVID-19 pandemic and the implementation of alternative technological solutions. In some countries, although national telehealth centers existed before the pandemic, the necessity of integrating telehealth use into national healthcare services worldwide has emerged due to the COVID-19 pandemic [33, 40].

With the pandemic and COVID-19, specific problems have arisen in the acute and chronic management of pulmonary diseases. International associations have issued specific position statements for individuals with pulmonary diseases. Alternative rehabilitation program models tailored to the crisis have been identified. Configurations such as online educational sessions and virtual exercise sessions via telephone and video calls have improved patient outcomes [40, 41].

During the pandemic, advancements in mobile technologies have emerged to control the outbreak. Mainly, developments and assessments related to criteria such as usability, functionality, ethical issues, security and privacy, user perception, design, information, and content have been made in mobile phone applications used for contact tracing [42].

Following the pandemic, residual functional deficits have emerged in patients with post-COVID syndrome. Due to limited timeframes and insufficient capacity in terms of equipment, workforce, and other services during this period, the development of urgent remote rehabilitation systems has become necessary. Telerehabilitation models have been developed using digital communication technologies [43].

During the pandemic, telerehabilitation systems have enabled discharged patients to continue their treatments and promote further recovery. These systems have ensured the continuity of therapy through assessments synchronously or asynchronously (with recorded and customized exercise plans) [44].

Telerehabilitation applications were organized for patients whose discharges were expedited after appropriate medical treatment post-discharge. Initially, follow-up and medical monitoring were provided using teleconference platforms, especially in the early stages after discharge. Electronic coding systems were established to categorize patients based on their needs post-discharge. Telerehabilitation programs incorporating the fundamental components of pulmonary rehabilitation programs were often adapted to pandemic circumstances by enhancing existing applications [43].

6.1.7 Conclusions

Pulmonary rehabilitation programs are vital in improving the quality of life and overall health outcomes of individuals with chronic respiratory conditions. The necessity of adapting healthcare services, including telerehabilitation systems, has become evident in mandatory situations where traditional methods, such as during the pandemic, cannot be applied and services adapting to technological advancements. Technological systems provide alternative solutions in all rehabilitation programs. Combining clinical rehabilitation services with the advantages of telerehabilitation systems or evaluating their effectiveness through conducted studies is recommended. Standardization and collaboration for these systems should be established with organizations and health and technology experts, and education and information support systems should be developed to eliminate disadvantages and limitations. Increasing the accessibility and suitability of systems, evaluating their long-term effects, providing support for security and privacy management, and improving them will result in remarkable effects of telerehabilitation systems in pulmonary rehabilitation.

6.2 Cardiac Rehabilitation

6.2.1 Introduction

Cardiac rehabilitation ensures that individuals with heart disease achieve as optimal a position as possible within society in terms of their physical, cognitive, and social health, allowing them to maintain an active lifestyle [45]. Following a cardiac event, the benefits of cardiac rehabilitation include reducing cardiovascular risk factors, improving quality of life by incorporating healthy behaviors into daily life, facilitating adherence to these behaviors, and promoting an active lifestyle. Cardiac rehabilitation is a significant component of cardiovascular disease management [46]. Cardiac rehabilitation programs are typically conducted in a center, with sessions occurring 2–3 times/week for up to 6 months, under the supervision of healthcare professionals [47]. Despite the significant benefits of cardiac rehabilitation programs, access to these programs is deficient, ranging from 15% to 30% of eligible individuals. In Belgium, for example, only 15–20% of patients with cardiovascular disease participate in outpatient cardiac rehabilitation programs (Phase II), and only 5% participate in long-term Phase III care interventions [48]. The main reasons for this include accessibility to these programs, distance to the service center, reluctance of participants to attend group exercise sessions, personal economic constraints, and uncertainty about the effectiveness of such programs. Accessibility inequality significantly impacts the prognosis of cardiac diseases [47]. Addressing this need becomes crucial, especially during the COVID-19 pandemic crisis, which has restricted access to hospitals and increased the risk of transmission [46].

Telerehabilitation (TR) may be an effective and safe alternative or complementary approach to center-based cardiac rehabilitation. It can help individuals with cardiac disease access supervised physical exercise in their homes or social environments. In TR programs, patient data, physical activity, blood pressure, electrocardiography (ECG) recordings, heart rate variability, oxygen saturation, and other relevant metrics are monitored and reported to healthcare professionals. Personalized feedback is provided at intervals to ensure an appropriate exercise program for the patient [47]. In recent years, telerehabilitation applications have become more widespread, driven by advancements in new information technologies and telemedical devices [49]. Decreases in Internet costs and increased presence of communication technologies in social life have facilitated the use of technology-based approaches to continue healthcare services both during hospitalization and after discharge. Moreover, the rising elderly population in developed societies and the consequent inadequacy of resources allocated by countries to public health have led to a search for new applications areas in healthcare [50]. Furthermore, the COVID-19 pandemic has further accelerated the use of telerehabilitation approaches, making them necessary during the pandemic [51]. In Turkey, as in the rest of the world, implementing cardiac telehealth approaches has gained momentum. Physiotherapists are developing and implementing expert approaches to cardiac telerehabilitation.

Cardiac rehabilitation is a multidisciplinary program aimed at achieving optimal physical, psychological, and functional status within the limitations of individuals affected by cardiovascular system impairment through exercise, behavior change, and education. The program includes educating patients and their families on the treatment, prevention, and recognition of cardiovascular disease, reducing or improving risk factors, addressing psychological factors that affect cardiac disease recovery, structured progressive physical activity under supervision in rehabilitation centers or home programs, and vocational counseling [52, 53].

It is noted that there is insufficient emphasis on the importance of primary prevention aimed at preventing the onset of cardiovascular disease. Cardiac rehabilitation mainly encompasses secondary prevention approaches based on early detection and prevention of cardiovascular disease progression. These approaches involve instilling lifestyle changes and providing education, counseling, and behavioral strategies for managing risk factors [52, 53].

In recent years, significant advancements have been made in understanding the natural course of many cardiac pathologies, yet heart disease continues to be the leading cause of mortality. This underscores the necessity of widespread implementation of cardiac rehabilitation within healthcare systems to reduce mortality and morbidity [54].

In recent years, cardiac rehabilitation has evolved into a multidisciplinary program encompassing activities ranging from simple monitoring program follow-up to safely returning to physical activities, postoperative patient care, optimization of medical treatment, nutrition counseling, smoking cessation, risk stratification, stress management, hypertension management, and control of diabetes or dyslipidemia. According to the World Health Organization, cardiac rehabilitation is the sum of activities necessary to positively influence the underlying causes of cardiac disease and provide the patient with the best possible physical, mental, and social conditions. Ultimately, patients can achieve a place in community life as possible through their efforts and actively participate in their own lives through rehabilitation [55].

6.2.2 Telehealth Approaches in Cardiac Rehabilitation

While modern healthcare systems offer significant opportunities to patients, they also face substantial challenges. Changing demographics, rapidly advancing medical technology, and regional issues in providing healthcare to low-density populations are among the most critical challenges. Additionally, increased life expectancy and a growing geriatric population lead to a growing need for the care and monitoring of individuals with chronic diseases and older individuals living at home [56].

The latest guidelines from the Centers for Disease Control and Prevention, developed by experts, recommend that all high-risk individuals, including those with cardiovascular risk factors, stay at home to limit exposure to COVID-19 and restrict direct contact between healthcare personnel and patients due to the high transmission rates of COVID-19. Therefore, especially during the COVID-19 pandemic, experts suggest taking intervention measures such as digital solutions and online healthcare services instead of face-to-face rehabilitation programs, which increase the risk of transmission [57].

Telehealth involves using information and communication technologies (ICTs) to improve health and healthcare-related activities. Advances in telehealth and telemedicine in cardiac rehabilitation have facilitated access to more elderly individuals and individuals with chronic diseases, addressing the increasing need for chronic disease treatment, reversing negative lifestyle changes, benefiting from advancements in modern medicine, addressing regional issues in providing healthcare to low-density populations, facilitating access to patient data and documents, and optimizing treatment while avoiding unnecessary interventions [56].

6.2.3 Challenges in the Implementation of Telehealth and Telemedicine

There are significant barriers to integrating telehealth approaches into daily clinical practice. These barriers include the weak and conflicting evidence base regarding the value of telehealth and telemedicine in managing various cardiovascular diseases. Priority is often given to technical advancements in the development of telehealth and telemedicine, while the needs and expectations of healthcare professionals and patients are inadequately met. Common platforms and connections between devices and systems used in telehealth approaches are often insufficient. Additionally, severe issues regarding patient information privacy and data security are reported. The most significant barriers to the widespread implementation of evidence-based tools in telehealth and telemedicine include equipment and setup costs, cost-effectiveness calculations, and regulatory gaps in the reimbursement of telehealth and telemedicine services [56].

Various alternative approaches to cardiac rehabilitation (CR) have been developed to promote its use and optimize its long-term effects [58]. Modern technological and telemedical advancements enable healthcare professionals to monitor patients remotely [59].

Implementing telehealth to provide CR services is a significant innovation in improving patient intake, selection, and access to rehabilitation [46, 56]. Implementing exercise programs through telehealth in CR is considered as effective as center-based CR programs in improving modifiable cardiovascular risk factors and functional capacity. Additionally, providing CR at home for patients unable to attend center-based programs offers the advantage of broader CR utilization [60].

Telehealth approaches that enable remote patient monitoring include prevention and lifestyle interventions, management of chronic diseases such as hypertension, diabetes mellitus, and heart failure, arrhythmia detection, and telerehabilitation [56].

6.2.3.1 Prevention and Lifestyle Interventions

Prevention approaches for cardiac diseases are considered the most important and economical intervention. Prevention approaches have the most significant potential impact in reducing the burden of cardiovascular disease. Monitoring cardiovascular risk factors through surveillance, education, psychological support, and interactive motivational devices has improved lifestyle and medical therapy adherence. As a result, individuals' metabolic risk factors decrease, and cardiovascular health improves through enhancing physical activity, promoting healthy eating, and smoking cessation. The widespread implementation of remote activity monitoring and personal data collection in preventing and managing chronic diseases is likely to have a significant impact on increasing patient compliance. Activity tracking with wearable devices provides substantial benefits, particularly in postoperative recovery in heart patients, pulmonary rehabilitation, and activity counseling for diabetes patients [56].

6.2.3.2 Telecare

Telecare is stated as an imaging method in cardiac patients. Telecare involves the transmission of symptoms, signs, and biological or physiological data from one location to another for interpretation and decision-making. Telecare includes the remote visualization of symptoms (such as chest pain, fatigue, shortness of breath, edema, etc.) and physiological data (such as heart rate, ECG, weight, and blood pressure) from external imaging devices or cardiovascular implantable electronic devices or implantable hemodynamic devices monitored at home [59].

The content of telecare includes teleassessment (active remote assessment), tele-support (e.g., supportive television by nurses, psychological support), teletherapy (interactive therapy), tele-coaching (support and instruction for treatment), teleconsultation, and telerehabilitation (TR). TR is supervised remote comprehensive cardiac rehabilitation and includes exercise training within telecare and tele-dentistry [59].

6.2.3.3 Telerehabilitation

The remote delivery of cardiac rehabilitation (CR) has long been studied as an alternative or adjunct intervention to overcome common barriers to CR participation, such as distance, transportation, or timing constraints [51]. The European Society of Cardiology guidelines consider cardiac telerehabilitation (CTR) as a valid alternative approach [58].

Recent advances in information and communication technologies have facilitated telerehabilitation's provision, monitoring, and guidance. The utilization of these technological innovations for delivering remote CR is termed telerehabilitation. Telerehabilitation allows patients to monitor their progress and receive objective feedback. Additionally, telerehabilitation can help patients develop self-management skills and support the maintenance of behavior change. It is observed that most telerehabilitation methods focus only on exercise training and physical activity components. However, the ideal approach is for telerehabilitation to encompass all the core components of CR tailored to the individual patient's risk factors [61].

The most commonly used telerehabilitation methods (teleconsultation, teletherapy, tele-mentoring, or tele-imaging) are delivered through electronic methods, mobile texting, or short messaging service (SMS). These methods are also implemented through video calling and instant messaging via social media platforms such as Viber™, Skype™, or FaceTime™ etc. [62].

With the increasing research on cardiac telerehabilitation approaches in recent years, these applications have become a focus of CR, particularly in the post-COVID era. In CTR, sections of the CR program are conducted in the patient's home environment using remote communication (e.g., web or mobile applications) and wearable devices (e.g., heart rate monitors, accelerometers) [58].

A meta-analysis reported that telerehabilitation for heart failure patients improved functional capacity and quality of life compared to usual care. Furthermore, various meta-analyses and systematic reviews have indicated that multidisciplinary or exercise-based cardiac telerehabilitation is as safe and effective as center-based CR [47, 63, 64].

6.2.4 Advantages of Telerehabilitation

TR's most significant advantages include providing greater privacy, allowing individuals to determine their own pace and timing, minimal travel/transportation barriers, higher patient independence, integration with remote monitoring, protection from viral infections, provision of core components at home, and being cost-effective [59].

6.2.4.1 Advantages from the Patient Perspective

The application of TR in familiar environments, namely at home, allows individuals to exercise independently, at their own pace, and at a chosen time. Real-time videoconferences (advanced telemonitoring systems) enable patients to continue rehabilitation if they encounter difficulties adhering to hospital-based programs. Eliminating transportation-related issues (time and cost savings) and enhancing patient independence while performing daily tasks are significant aspects [59].

6.2.4.2 Advantages from the Healthcare Professional Perspective

TR offers the opportunity to treat more patients and combines patient monitoring with tele-imaging, increasing control for patient compliance [59].

6.2.4.3 Advantages for the Healthcare System

New equipment and technology become rapidly accessible and provide cost-effectiveness. For example, replacing parts or adding to existing care depends on usage [59].

6.2.5 Telerehabilitation Systems

6.2.5.1 Heart Rate Monitoring

Data obtained through exercise logs and heart rate monitors are recorded on a computer. The telemedicine team communicates with patients weekly via telephone or email and prepares reports on their progress. Patients are required to report heart rate readings and exercise logs every 4–6 weeks [58]. Mobile technologies, especially smartphones, are also increasingly used for heart rate monitoring [64]. Smart et al. conducted studies on patients with chronic heart failure who used exercise training at home with heart rate monitoring and exercise logs, providing feedback on their progress. As a result, the remote monitoring approach can be used to monitor compliance with home exercise training [65].

6.2.5.2 Transtelephonic Electrocardiographic Monitoring

The system is installed in a public gym with telephonic electrocardiographic monitoring kits. If concerning symptoms are noticed during monitoring, the patient's 12-lead EKG is taken and transmitted in real-time via regular telephone lines by expert trainers. Healthcare personnel in the telecare unit evaluate the data sent. If a cardiologist deems it necessary to intervene after a final assessment, they contact the exercise trainer to provide instructions [66].

6.2.5.3 Remote Exercise Training Device for Tele-Electrocardiogram Monitoring and Supervision

Equipment in the system is adjusted according to the patient's characteristics. The system includes a device for EKG recording, blood pressure measurement, body weight machines, a cell phone, and a cell phone-based data transmission set. The patient's current condition and medication are recorded before training. Resting EKG, blood pressure, and weight data are sent to the monitoring center. If no contraindication is detected, the training program begins. Each set includes the patient's individualized training session, exercise duration, breaks, and timing of EKG recording. After the training session, if there are no adverse symptoms, the EKG recording is sent to the monitoring center for evaluation. Based on the data, consultants determine the training workload. The monitoring center collects and evaluates patients' health data to create a follow-up report [59].

6.2.5.4 Real-Time Electrocardiographic and Voice Transtelephonic Monitoring of Cardiac Rehabilitation

The application includes a real-time transtelephonic electrocardiographic transmitter, a headset with headphones, and a microphone for patients. Up to four patients are monitored simultaneously, and conference phone calls are made. This supports group interaction among participants and assists monitoring staff in directing teaching and group therapy sessions [59].

6.2.5.5 Remote Monitoring of Physical Activity Using Motion Sensors

Recently, two motion sensors, accelerometers, and pedometers, have been commonly used. The accelerometer collects data to assess and measure any movement related to physical activity. It also provides numerical data determining the intensity, frequency, and duration of physical activity by offering continuous and continuous monitoring. Pedometers measure the number of steps taken in a day, enabling the calculation of distance covered and energy consumption values [59].

6.2.5.6 Using Game Systems for Rehabilitation

Exercise-based gaming systems, such as Nintendo Wii Fit, have been developed for rehabilitation purposes, including active video games. The system transmits real-time data collected via Bluetooth to the Wii console. Nicholson et al. applied unsupervised Nintendo Wii Fit balance training to elderly adults for 6 weeks, three sessions per week, and 30 min/session. As a result, unsupervised Wii balance games are reported to be a valuable approach for improving balance in independent elderly adults [67].

In a case study by Klompstra et al., a 74-year-old patient with chronic heart failure tracked daily physical activity using Nintendo Wii Fit for 12 weeks. As a result, it was reported that the patient's daily energy expenditure, exercise capacity, and exercise motivation increased [68].

The "Exergaming" approach, especially with the Wii® platform, promises to be a promising application for engaging in physical activity. This approach combines virtual reality-based activities with video games and exercise. The interaction of specialized exercises with games in Exergaming benefits patients' physical fitness. Additionally, in patients, particularly those comprising most of the young population, exercising is vital in increasing physical activity, especially in patient motivation [59, 69].

6.2.5.7 Mobile Health Technologies (mHealth)

Mobile technologies based on smartphones, smartwatches, and fitness program trackers (fitness trackers) provide objective physical activity monitoring. They offer detailed information on the type, intensity, and frequency of physical activity and assist in implementing behavior change techniques [70]. With mHealth technologies, medical approaches are renewed by enabling increased patient participation, monitoring, social support, and healthcare services. In cardiac rehabilitation, mHealth technologies include smartphone applications, wearable devices, and handheld devices, offering real-time tracking of numerous necessary physiological measurements and other parameters [18].

Applications are available for smartphones and personal digital assistants to measure different movements. Some types of cell phones have an accelerometer function, while others have health diary software that collects data on the patient's physiological condition and medical information. Healthcare professionals can use web portals to set personal goals for patients and assess the progress of those involved in telerehabilitation programs. Educational multimedia programs can be sent to participants and monitored [59].

The use of smartphones has increased significantly. Their procurement, portability, user-friendliness, relatively low prices, wireless connectivity, extensive computing capabilities, and comprehensive memories make them useful for healthcare services. Smartphones are generally connected to a mobile sensor or medical device to measure vital signs [65].

6.2.6 Focus Points of Telerehabilitation

Despite its numerous benefits, key areas need to be addressed to provide solutions. These include the need for digital literacy, the inadequacy of reimbursement in the healthcare system, the necessity for integration in electronic medical records, reduced face-to-face interactions, data security and privacy concerns, lack of legal frameworks, and limited social interaction [51].

6.2.7 Limitations of Telerehabilitation

6.2.7.1 Limitations from the Perspective of Patients

Technological skills, addressing potential issues, and the lack of face-to-face interaction with healthcare personnel and other patients are limitations. Despite the increasing access to the Internet in today's society, the likelihood of cardiovascular patients having access to and utilizing these technologies decreases due to factors such as advanced age, lower education levels, and residing in rural areas.

However, between 2013 and 2016, it is known that Internet usage in Canada increased by approximately 25% among individuals aged 65–74 and by over 40% among those aged 75 and older. A study conducted in 2009, specifically on heart patients, revealed that two-thirds of hospitalized patients had Internet access at home, and more than half of these patients accessed the Internet daily. Smartphone ownership rates have also increased in these age groups, with over a third of individuals owning smartphones. It is anticipated that as individuals who use these digital technologies in their 50s and 60s continue to age, the digital divide related to age will likely diminish over time [71].

6.2.7.2 Limitations from the Perspective of Experts

There is no "applied" real-time interaction [59]. Some studies indicate minor side effects (such as angina, sweating, ankle pain, etc.) in cardiac telerehabilitation (TR). In emergencies like these, immediate medical assistance cannot be provided [47]. Additionally, conducting telephone-based applications for cardiac rehabilitation education groups is more challenging [59].

6.2.7.3 Limitations Within the Healthcare System

Issues with reimbursement, lack of legal principles, and absence of a comprehensive telemedical integration system are reported [59].

6.2.8 Telerehabilitation with Exercise Training

Telerehabilitation approaches can support long-term adherence to physical activity recommendations in Phase II and III CR. Frederix et al. in 2015 used telerehabilitation in addition to standard CR. Text messaging and accelerometer monitoring were used for exercise tracking in telerehabilitation content. Significant improvements in physical fitness and quality of life were reported after the 6-month telerehabilitation program [72]. Additionally, in the study by Frederix et al. in 2017, individualized exercise prescriptions were provided to patients through CR and telerehabilitation, and patients were given the task of self-monitoring with accelerometers. The study concluded that the health benefits were sustained, and the cost was advantageous for up to 2 years [73].

In a study by Avila et al., a short-term home-based Phase III CR exercise program was guided remotely. Patients were instructed to use a smartwatch to record their physical activities and upload this data to an online web application. The study concluded that short-term home-based telerehabilitation was as beneficial as long-term center-based training and achieved similar effects on physical activity and exercise capacity [74].

Piotrowicz et al. conducted a long-term telerehabilitation study for heart failure (HF) patients. The telerehabilitation program included three training approaches: endurance aerobic Nordic walking training, respiratory muscle training, and light resistance and strength exercises. Tele-monitoring included tele-ECG visualization and supervised exercise training using a remote device, data transmission via mobile phones, and medical data control. The study concluded that the telerehabilitation intervention was effective over 9 weeks (1 week in the hospital and 8 weeks at home), significantly improving peak oxygen consumption and quality of life [75].

Kraal et al. compared a 12-week center-based exercise training in Phase II CR with a 12-week home-based exercise training. The study utilized coaching interventions, including strategies for behavior change, to maintain adherence to a healthy lifestyle and improve long-term effects, using tele-guidance with tele-monitoring. Patients in the home exercise program used a wearable heart rate monitor to record physical activity data uploaded to the Internet. Progress was monitored weekly by the therapist through telephone calls. The study concluded that home-based tele-guided intervention was equally effective as center-based training regarding physical fitness, physical activity level, and health-related quality of life [76]. Additionally, a study reported that home-based exercise training resulted in higher patient satisfaction than center-based training and had lower costs than center-based education [77].

Maddison et al. evaluated the effectiveness of a personalized 12-week exercise program for CAD patients using a smartphone and a wearable sensor attached to the chest, monitoring and educating patients through a remote CR platform. The sensor provided information on heart and respiratory rates, single-lead ECG, and accelerometer data. An objective physical activity assessment was conducted using an accelerometer worn on the waist for seven consecutive days. The authors showed that remote CR increased access to rehabilitation, provided unique participant preferences, and was a practical and cost-effective intervention that could improve overall CR usage rates [78].

Rawstorn et al. compared the effects and costs of an innovative smartphone cardiac rehabilitation-assisted self-management (SCRAM) intervention with usual care CR in a 24-week randomized controlled trial. The study involved 220 adults in two phases. The first phase included 12 weeks of real-time remote exercise management with exercise physiologist coaching. The second phase consisted of a 12-week data-driven, non-real-time remote coaching program via telephone. SCRAM included a wearable sensor, an Android-based smartphone in the mobile health platform, and a CR web application for health professionals compatible with mobile and desktop web browsers. The exercise program was personalized under the supervision of an exercise physiologist, and exercise performance was measured using a smartphone application and a wearable sensor. The intervention impacted cardiac and all-cause mortality outcomes, providing positive and valuable evidence regarding acceptability and cost-effectiveness [79].

Serón et al. will conduct an effective (non-inferiority), pragmatic, multicenter, parallel-group (1:1), prospective, randomized, double-anonymized, endpoint evaluation clinical trial. The study will randomize 308 patients with coronary artery disease to hybrid or standard rehabilitation programs. The hybrid CR program includes ten supervised exercise sessions, individualized lifestyle counseling by a physiotherapist, and an unsupervised program via text messages and phone calls 4–6 weeks later. The supervised program consists of 4–6 weeks of aerobic and resistance training led by a physiotherapist. Exercise sessions start at 10 min and increase to 60 min. The exercise intensity will be moderate. Suppose the hybrid model is shown to be effective. In that case, it is expected to be a feasible CR program for patients and the healthcare system to improve cardiovascular health outcomes and cost-effectiveness [80].

Claes et al. applied the Health for Physical Activity (PATHway) platform developed to increase adherence to new care approaches from remotely delivered telerehabilitation programs in their study. The PATHway includes a comprehensive, Internet-connected, sensor-based home CR platform. It contains personalized exercise programs (exercise classes and exercise games) monitored by personalized heart rate, forming the basis of a customized lifestyle intervention program. This pilot study aims to provide insight into changes in the patient's health status and the system's effectiveness [81].

Most studies indicate comparable exercise capacity and quality of life results between center-based CR and telerehabilitation. However, the impact of telerehabilitation on recurrent events, re-hospitalizations, and mortality in patients with CAD and CHF is rarely investigated. Additionally, there is a lack of studies evaluating the effects of telerehabilitation on CR participation rates [51, 76]. Furthermore, Scherrenberg et al. noted that most studies focus on Phase II or Phase III CR, with telerehabilitation studies rarely targeting Phase I CR [51].

6.2.9 Smoking Cessation with Telehealth

Smoking is considered a critical modifiable risk factor that should be targeted for cessation as part of primary and secondary prevention programs for cardiovascular disease. Various technological approaches such as telephone counseling, video counseling, Internet-based interventions, text messaging, or mobile applications are utilized to provide remote guidance for smoking cessation [51].

6.2.10 Patient Education with Telerehabilitation

Education in cardiac disease is essential in secondary prevention and cardiac rehabilitation (CR) programs. According to the American Heart Association's 2018 report, limited health literacy is positively associated with patient morbidity, mortality, healthcare utilization, and costs [51]. Additionally, studies have found that inadequate health literacy is associated with worse overall health status, increased risk of hospital readmission, and mortality [82]. Education in CR programs can reduce cardiovascular events and improve health-related quality of life [51].

Remote education is delivered through various means such as telephone, email, text messaging, social media, or video counseling. The advantage of the education approach is easy and quick access and the ability of healthcare professionals to deliver necessary information to patients at regular intervals [51]. Implementation of telephone support in CR programs has been shown to reduce anxiety and depression, improve blood pressure, and assist in smoking cessation [83]. Experts also find the education approach in CR advantageous in terms of cost [51]. Desteghe et al. set up an online education platform to educate patients with atrial fibrillation (AF) about their condition. This approach was considered effective, showing lasting impact for up to 12 weeks after the procedure [84]. Additionally, a lifestyle-focused text messaging service has significantly improved reducing risk factors for coronary artery disease (CAD) in patients with diabetes mellitus (DM) [85]. Multiple strategies can be applied to remote education in cardiac rehabilitation. Among these methods, telephone counseling and written messaging appear suitable due to their ease of setup and implementation [51].

6.2.11 Telerehabilitation Approaches Used in Phase II CR

It is noted that home-based cardiac telerehabilitation (TR) approaches are mainly delivered through web-based platforms and smartphone applications in Phase II CR. Telemonitoring devices such as pedometers, accelerometers, and heart rate monitors support physical activity. Additionally, complementary communication approaches such as text messages, phone calls, video calls, and emails are used for communication between participants and the intervention team. Some studies encompass critical components of secondary prevention, including managing cardiovascular disease (CVD) risk factors, physical activity, smoking cessation, medication adherence, and stress management. However, it is observed that some studies focus solely on physical activity [86].

References

1. Soriano JB, Kendrick PJ, Paulson KR, et al. Prevalence and attributable health burden of chronic respiratory diseases, 1990–2017: a systematic analysis for the Global Burden of Disease Study 2017. Lancet Respir Med. 2020;8:585–96.
2. Ergan M, Başkurt Z. Pulmoner Hastaliklard Telerehabílítasyon. SDÜ Tıp Fakültesi Derg. 2021;28:361–5.
3. Spruit MA, Singh SJ, Garvey C, et al. An official American Thoracic Society/European Respiratory Society statement: key concepts and advances in pulmonary rehabilitation. Am J Respir Crit Care Med. 2013;188(8):e13–64. https://doi.org/10.1164/rccm.201309-1634ST.
4. Collins EG, Langbein WE, Fehr L, O'Connell S, Jelinek C, Hagarty E, Edwards L, Reda D, Tobin MJ, Laghi F. Can ventilation-feedback training augment exercise tolerance in patients with chronic obstructive pulmonary disease? Am J Respir Crit Care Med. 2008;177:844–52.

5. Chodzko-Zajko WJ, Proctor DN, Fiatarone Singh MA, Minson CT, Nigg CR, Salem GJ, Skinner JS. Exercise and physical activity for older adults. Med Sci Sports Exerc. 2009;41:1510–30.
6. Fischer MJ, Scharloo M, Abbink JJ, van 't Hul AJ, van Ranst D, Rudolphus A, Weinman J, Rabe KF, Kaptein AA. Drop-out and attendance in pulmonary rehabilitation: the role of clinical and psychosocial variables. Respir Med. 2009;103:1564–71.
7. Milner SC, Boruff JT, Beaurepaire C, Ahmed S, Janaudis-Ferreira T. Rate of, and barriers and enablers to, pulmonary rehabilitation referral in COPD: a systematic scoping review. Respir Med. 2018;137:103–14.
8. Zheng J, Hou M, Liu L, Wang X. Knowledge structure and emerging trends of telerehabilitation in recent 20 years: a bibliometric analysis via CiteSpace. Front Public Health. 2022;10:1–16.
9. WHO. Global diffusion of eHealth: making universal health coverage achievable. Report of the Third Global Survey on eHealth. WHO; 2016.
10. Kairy D, Lehoux P, Vincent C, Visintin M. A systematic review of clinical outcomes, clinical process, healthcare utilization and costs associated with telerehabilitation. Disabil Rehabil. 2009;31:427–47.
11. Seron P, Oliveros MJ, Gutierrez-Arias R, et al. Effectiveness of telerehabilitation in physical therapy: a rapid overview. Phys Ther. 2021;101:1–18.
12. Selzler AM, Wald J, Sedeno M, Jourdain T, Janaudis-Ferreira T, Goldstein R, Bourbeau J, Stickland MK. Telehealth pulmonary rehabilitation: a review of the literature and an example of a nationwide initiative to improve the accessibility of pulmonary rehabilitation. Chron Respir Dis. 2018;15:41–7.
13. Cox NS, Dal Corso S, Hansen H, McDonald CF, Hill CJ, Zanaboni P, Alison JA, O'Halloran P, Macdonald H, Holland AE. Telerehabilitation for chronic respiratory disease. Cochrane Database Syst Rev. 2021;1(1):CD013040. https://doi.org/10.1002/14651858.CD013040.pub2.
14. Hwang R, Bruning J, Morris N, Mandrusiak A, Russell T. A systematic review of the effects of telerehabilitation in patients with cardiopulmonary diseases. J Cardiopulm Rehabil Prev. 2015;35:380–9.
15. Tsai LLY, McNamara RJ, Moddel C, Alison JA, McKenzie DK, McKeough ZJ. Home-based telerehabilitation via real-time videoconferencing improves endurance exercise capacity in patients with COPD: the randomized controlled TeleR study. Respirology. 2017;22:699–707.
16. Paneroni M, Colombo F, Papalia A, Colitta A, Borghi G, Saleri M, Cabiaglia A, Azzalini E, Vitacca M. Is telerehabilitation a safe and viable option for patients with COPD? A feasibility study. COPD J Chronic Obstr Pulm Dis. 2015;12:217–25.
17. Ryu S. Book review: mHealth: new horizons for health through mobile technologies: based on the findings of the second global survey on eHealth (Global observatory for eHealth series, volume 3). Healthc Inform Res. 2012;18:231.
18. MacKinnon GE, Brittain EL. Mobile health technologies in cardiopulmonary disease. Chest. 2020;157:654–64.
19. Spring B, Pellegrini C, McFadden HG, Pfammatter AF, Stump TK, Siddique J, King AC, Hedeker D. Multicomponent mHealth intervention for large, sustained change in multiple diet and activity risk behaviors: the make better choices 2 randomized controlled trial. J Med Internet Res. 2018;20:1–13.
20. Godino JG, Merchant G, Norman GJ, Donohue MC, Marshall SJ, Fowler JH, Calfas KJ, Huang JS. Using social and mobile tools for weight loss in overweight and obese young adults (project SMART): a 2-year parallel group randomized controlled trial acquisition, analysis, or interpretation of data: HHS public access. Lancet Diabetes Endocrinol. 2016;4:747–55.
21. Martin SS, Feldman DI, Blumenthal RS, et al. mActive: a randomized clinical trial of an automated mHealth intervention for physical activity promotion. J Am Heart Assoc. 2015;4:1–9.
22. Spielmanns M, Boeselt T, Huber S, et al. Impact of a smartphone application (KAIA COPD app) in combination with activity monitoring as a maintenance program following pulmonary rehabilitation in COPD: the protocol for the AMOPUR study, an international, multicenter, parallel group, randomized, controlled study. Trials. 2020;21:1–13.

23. Burkow TM, Vognild LK, Johnsen E, Bratvold A, Risberg MJ. Promoting exercise training and physical activity in daily life: a feasibility study of a virtual group intervention for behaviour change in COPD. BMC Med Inform Decis Mak. 2018;18:1–13.
24. Bao Y, Wang C, Xu H, Lai Y, Yan Y, Ma Y, Yu T, Wu Y. Effects of an mHealth intervention for pulmonary tuberculosis self-management based on the integrated theory of health behavior change: randomized controlled trial. JMIR Public Heal Surveill. 2022;8(7):e34277. https://doi.org/10.2196/34277.
25. Keating A, Lee A, Holland AE. What prevents people with chronic obstructive pulmonary disease from attending pulmonary rehabilitation? A systematic review. Chron Respir Dis. 2011;8:89–99.
26. Cox NS, Oliveira CC, Lahham A, Holland AE. Pulmonary rehabilitation referral and participation are commonly influenced by environment, knowledge, and beliefs about consequences: a systematic review using the Theoretical Domains Framework. J Physiother. 2017;63:84–93.
27. Johnston CL, Maxwell LJ, Maguire GP, Alison JA. How prepared are rural and remote health care practitioners to provide evidence-based management for people with chronic lung disease? Aust J Rural Health. 2012;20:200–7.
28. Cox NS, Khor YH. Telerehabilitation in pulmonary diseases. Curr Opin Pulm Med. 2023;29:313–21.
29. Aragaki D, Luo J, Weiner E, Zhang G, Darvish B. Cardiopulmonary telerehabilitation. Phys Med Rehabil Clin N Am. 2021;32:263–76.
30. Jones AW, Taylor A, Gowler H, O'Kelly N, Ghosh S, Bridle C. Systematic review of interventions to improve patient uptake and completion of pulmonary rehabilitation in COPD. ERJ Open Res. 2017;3(1):00089-2016. https://doi.org/10.1183/23120541.00089-2016.
31. Havran MA, Bidelspach DE. Virtual physical therapy and telerehabilitation. Phys Med Rehabil Clin N Am. 2021;32:419–28.
32. Chow CK, Ariyarathna N, Islam SMS, Thiagalingam A, Redfern J. mHealth in cardiovascular health care. Hear Lung Circ. 2016;25:802–7.
33. Jácome C, Marques A, Oliveira A, Rodrigues LV, Sanches I. Pulmonary telerehabilitation: an international call for action. Pulmonology. 2020;26:335–7.
34. Vitacca M, Kaymaz D, Lanini B, et al. Non-invasive ventilation during cycle exercise training in patients with chronic respiratory failure on long-term ventilatory support: a randomized controlled trial. Respirology. 2018;23:182–9.
35. Nuara A, Fabbri-Destro M, Scalona E, Lenzi SE, Rizzolatti G, Avanzini P. Telerehabilitation in response to constrained physical distance: an opportunity to rethink neurorehabilitative routines. J Neurol. 2022;269:627–38.
36. Seidman Z, McNamara R, Wootton S, Leung R, Spencer L, Dale M, Dennis S, McKeough Z. People attending pulmonary rehabilitation demonstrate a substantial engagement with technology and willingness to use telerehabilitation: a survey. J Physiother. 2017;63:175–81.
37. Wilde LJ, Sewell L, Percy C, Ward G, Clark C. What are the experiences of people with COPD using activity monitors?: a qualitative scoping review. COPD J Chronic Obstr Pulm Dis. 2022;19:88–98.
38. Bentley CL, Powell L, Potter S, et al. The use of a smartphone app and an activity tracker to promote physical activity in the management of chronic obstructive pulmonary disease: randomized controlled feasibility study. JMIR Mhealth Uhealth. 2020;8:1–21.
39. Tsutsui M, Gerayeli F, Sin DD. Pulmonary rehabilitation in a post-covid-19 world: telerehabilitation as a new standard in patients with COPD. Int J COPD. 2021;16:379–91.
40. Wen J, Milne S, Sin DD. Pulmonary rehabilitation in a postcoronavirus disease 2019 world: feasibility, challenges, and solutions. Curr Opin Pulm Med. 2022;28:152–61.
41. Bhutani M, Hernandez P, Bourbeau J, et al. Key highlights of the Canadian Thoracic Society's position statement on the optimization of COPD management during the coronavirus disease 2019 pandemic. Chest. 2020;158:869–72.
42. Chidambaram S, Erridge S, Kinross J, Purkayastha S. Observational study of UK mobile health apps for COVID-19. Lancet Digit Health. 2020;2:e388–90.

43. Salawu A, Green A, Crooks MG, Brixey N, Ross DH, Sivan M. A proposal for multidisciplinary tele-rehabilitation in the assessment and rehabilitation of COVID-19 survivors. Int J Environ Res Public Health. 2020;17:1–13.
44. Sheehy LM. Considerations for postacute rehabilitation for survivors of COVID-19. JMIR Public Heal Surveill. 2020;6:1–8.
45. Hillegass EA, Steven SH. Cardiopulmonary physical therapy. 2nd ed. Philadephia: W.B. Saunders; 2001.
46. Neubeck L. Telehealth-based cardiac rehabilitation: a solution to the problem of access? Eur J Prev Cardiol. 2015;22(8):957–8.
47. Cavalheiro AH, et al. Effectiveness of tele-rehabilitation programs in heart failure: a systematic review and meta-analysis. Health Services Insights. 2021;14:11786329211021668.
48. De Vos C, et al. Participating or not in a cardiac rehabilitation programme: factors influencing a patient's decision. Eur J Prevent Cardiol. 2013;20(2):341–8.
49. Peretti A, et al. Telerehabilitation: review of the state-of-the-art and areas of application. JMIR Rehabil Assist Technol. 2017;4(2):e7511.
50. Agostini M, et al. Telerehabilitation and recovery of motor function: a systematic review and meta-analysis. J Telemed Telecare. 2015;21(4):202–13.
51. Scherrenberg M, et al. The future is now: a call for action for cardiac telerehabilitation in the COVID-19 pandemic from the secondary prevention and rehabilitation section of the European Association of Preventive Cardiology. Eur J Prev Cardiol. 2021;28(5):524–40.
52. Giannuzzi P, et al. Secondary prevention through cardiac rehabilitation: position paper of the Working Group on Cardiac Rehabilitation and Exercise Physiology of the European Society of Cardiology. Eur Heart J. 2003;24(13):1273–8.
53. Mampuya WM. Cardiac rehabilitation past, present and future: an overview. Cardiovasc Diagn Ther. 2012;2(1):38.
54. Sari DM, Wijaya LCG. Cardiac rehabilitation via telerehabilitation in COVID-19 pandemic situation. Egypt Heart J. 2021;73(1):1–9.
55. Report of the World Health Organization Expert Committee on Disability Prevention and Rehabilitation. Rehabilitation after cardiovascular disease, with special emphasis on developing countries. Geneva: World Health Organization; 1993.
56. Saner H, van der Velde E. eHealth in cardiovascular medicine: a clinical update. Eur J Prevent Cardiol. 2016;23(2_Suppl):5–12.
57. Rutkowski S. Management challenges in chronic obstructive pulmonary disease in the COVID-19 pandemic: telehealth and virtual reality. J Clin Med. 2021;10(6):1261.
58. Vromen T, et al. Novel advances in cardiac rehabilitation: position paper from the Working Group on Preventive Cardiology and Cardiac Rehabilitation of the Netherlands Society of Cardiology. Neth Hear J. 2021;29:479–85.
59. Piotrowicz E, et al. Telerehabilitation in heart failure patients: the evidence and the pitfalls. Int J Cardiol. 2016;220:408–13.
60. Rawstorn JC, et al. Telehealth exercise-based cardiac rehabilitation: a systematic review and meta-analysis. Heart. 2016;102(15):1183–92.
61. Frederix I, Vanhees L, Dendale P, et al. A review of telerehabilitation for cardiac patients. J Telemed Telecare. 2015;21:45–53.
62. Leochico CD, et al. Challenges to the emergence of telerehabilitation in a developing country: a systematic review. Front Neurol. 2020;11:1007.
63. Huang K, Liu W, He D, et al. Telehealth interventions versus center-based cardiac rehabilitation of coronary artery disease: a systematic review and meta-analysis. Eur J Prev Cardiol. 2015;22:959–71.
64. De Ridder B, et al. Smartphone apps using photoplethysmography for heart rate monitoring: meta-analysis. JMIR Cardiol. 2018;2(1):e8802.
65. Smart N, Haluska B, Jeffriess L, et al. Predictors of sustained response to exercise training in patients with chronic heart failure: a telemonitoring study. Am Heart J. 2005;150:1240–7.
66. Kouidi E, et al. Transtelephonic electrocardiographic monitoring of an outpatient cardiac rehabilitation programme. Clin Rehabil. 2006;20(12):1100–4.

67. Nicholson VP, et al. Six weeks of unsupervised Nintendo Wii fit gaming is effective at improving balance in independent older adults. J Aging Phys Act. 2015;23(1):153–8.
68. Klompstra LV, Jaarsma T, Strömberg A. An in-depth, longitudinal examination of the daily physical activity of a patient with heart failure using a Nintendo Wii at home: a case report. J Rehabil Med. 2013;45(6):599–602.
69. Soares D, Magalhaes S, Viamonte S. Home-based programs and application of new technologies in cardiac rehabilitation. Int J Phys Med Rehabil. 2013;1:158. https://doi.org/10.4172/2329-9096.100015.
70. Meinhart F, et al. Mobile technologies to promote physical activity during cardiac rehabilitation: a scoping review. Sensors. 2021;21(1):65.
71. Lear SA. The delivery of cardiac rehabilitation using communications technologies: the "virtual" cardiac rehabilitation program. Can J Cardiol. 2018;34(10):S278–83.
72. Mayer CJ, et al. Peer reviewed: developing a Telephone Assessment of Physical Activity (TAPA) questionnaire for older adults. Prev Chronic Dis. 2008;5:1.
73. Frederix I, et al. Medium-term effectiveness of a comprehensive internet-based and patient-specific telerehabilitation program with text messaging support for cardiac patients: randomized controlled trial. J Med Internet Res. 2015;17:e4799.
74. Avila A, et al. Home-based exercise with telemonitoring guidance in patients with coronary artery disease: does it improve long-term physical fitness? Eur J Prev Cardiol. 2020;27(4):367–77.
75. Piotrowicz E, et al. Effects of a 9-week hybrid comprehensive telerehabilitation program on long-term outcomes in patients with heart failure: the telerehabilitation in Heart Failure Patients (TELEREH-HF) randomized clinical trial. JAMA Cardiol. 2020;5(3):300–8.
76. Kraal JJ, et al. Effects of home-based training with telemonitoring guidance in low to moderate risk patients entering cardiac rehabilitation: short-term results of the FIT@ home study. Eur J Prevent Cardiol. 2014;21(2_Suppl):26–31.
77. Kraal JJ, et al. Clinical and cost-effectiveness of home-based cardiac rehabilitation compared to conventional, centre-based cardiac rehabilitation: results of the FIT@ Home study. Eur J Prev Cardiol. 2017;24(12):1260–73.
78. Maddison R, et al. Effects and costs of real-time cardiac telerehabilitation: randomised controlled non-inferiority trial. Heart. 2019;105(2):122–9.
79. Rawstorn JC, et al. Smartphone cardiac rehabilitation, assisted self-management versus usual care: protocol for a multicenter randomized controlled trial to compare effects and costs among people with coronary heart disease. JMIR Res Protoc. 2020;9(1):e15022.
80. Serón P, et al. Hybrid cardiac rehabilitation trial (HYCARET): protocol of a randomised, multicentre, non-inferiority trial in South America. BMJ Open. 2019;9(10):e031213.
81. Claes J, et al. PATHway I: design and rationale for the investigation of the feasibility, clinical effectiveness and cost-effectiveness of a technology-enabled cardiac rehabilitation platform. BMJ Open. 2017;7(6):e016781.
82. Sentell T, et al. The influence of community and individual health literacy on self-reported health status. J Gen Intern Med. 2014;29(2):298–304.
83. Kotb A, Hsieh S, Wells GA. The effect of telephone support interventions on coronary artery disease (CAD) patient outcomes during cardiac rehabilitation: a systematic review and meta-analysis. PLoS One. 2014;9(5):e96581.
84. Desteghe L, et al. Effectiveness and usability of an online tailored education platform for atrial fibrillation patients undergoing a direct current cardioversion or pulmonary vein isolation. Int J Cardiol. 2018;272:123–9.
85. Haider R, et al. Effect of lifestyle focused text messaging on risk factor modification in patients with diabetes and coronary heart disease: a sub-analysis of the TEXT ME study. Diabetes Res Clin Pract. 2019;153:184–90.
86. Ramachandran HJ, et al. Effectiveness of home-based cardiac telerehabilitation as an alternative to phase 2 cardiac rehabilitation of coronary heart disease: a systematic review and meta-analysis. Eur J Prev Cardiol. 2022;29(7):1017–43.

Teleassessment Methods in Pediatric Rehabilitation

7

Ozden Gokcek

7.1 First Section

7.1.1 The Importance of Rehabilitation Practices in Children's Health and Diseases

Survival rates have increased since the 1990s. However, up to 50% of extremely low birth weight babies, who are among the high-risk babies, have disabilities such as neuromotor developmental delays, including cerebral palsy, loss of sensory perception and motor control, learning difficulties, attention, and behavior problems [1–3]. It is important for child health because high brain plasticity in infancy is at its highest level from approximately 2 months before term to approximately 6 months after term [4].

Early physiotherapy and rehabilitation practices have been shown to significantly affect neural proliferation and plasticity in the brain during the period of active synaptogenesis in early infancy. It has been determined that this approach effectively identifies and addresses children's physiological and anatomical deficiencies, promotes sensory development and functional movement, and helping them achieve the highest possible level of independence in cognitive, psychological, and social terms [5]. In addition, regular physiotherapy and rehabilitation practices play an important role in increasing the functionality and participation in daily life activities of disabled individuals and children and preventing complications [6, 7].

However, rehabilitation services were seriously disrupted during the pandemic process [8, 9]. It was determined that the interruption of the rehabilitation service negatively affected the quality of life of the children by disrupting the meeting of the child's therapy needs and that the parents faced difficulties regarding this issue [6, 9].

O. Gokcek (✉)
Department of Physiotherapy and Rehabilitation, Health Science Faculty, Ege University, İzmir, Turkey
e-mail: ozden.gokcek@ege.edu.tr

F. Özden et al. (eds.), *Telerehabilitation*, TELe-Health,
https://doi.org/10.1007/978-3-031-69080-8_7

Studies have reported that the rehabilitation services received by children with neurodevelopmental disorders were disrupted during the COVID-19 pandemic period [6, 10]. The COVID-19 pandemic has led to the widespread use of telerehabilitation in healthcare. This has provided therapists with the opportunity to monitor children and continue family-centered and home-based treatment services for children with special needs [11].

7.1.2 Background of Telerehabilitation

Telehealth applications have experienced significant growth in recent years due to the convenience of receiving services from the patient's home, resulting in time and cost savings, easy access to rehabilitation services, and the ability to provide long-term patient follow-up [12].

Telehealth utilizes electronic information and telecommunication technologies, such as smartphones and mobile wireless devices, to support clinical health care, patient education, public health, and management [13].

Telerehabilitation, a subfield of telehealth, involves the clinical application of counseling, preventive, diagnostic, and treatment services using telecommunications technology [13, 14]. Telerehabilitation services allow remote patient interaction, enabling remote examination, diagnosis, and treatment [15].

Telerehabilitation technologies include image-based, sensor-based, virtual reality, and virtual environment categories. Videoconferencing platforms are used for image-based telerehabilitation and modules such as counseling, physical evaluation, and training. Sensor-based telerehabilitation involves monitoring and evaluating body movements [16].

This method offers an advantage in achieving the therapist's goals in the home environment, assessing the parents' conditions, identifying the children's rehabilitation needs, and understanding their priorities [17].

7.1.3 Teleassessment Methods in Pediatric

7.1.3.1 5DT 5 Ultra Glove

The evaluation method in telerehabilitation involves an elastic glove with fiber optic sensors in each of the five fingers to detect changes in finger position. The performance of the gloved hand is monitored by the evaluator via a monitor with an internet connection. This sensor glove can measure hand function, grip strength, and range of motion [18].

7.1.3.2 TelereHUB-CHILD

TelereHUB-CHILD is an online information platform designed in collaboration with pediatric rehabilitation professionals, patients, and families. The TelereHUB-CHILD platform comprises four sections: Tele-Treatments, patient/family information, Tele-Evaluations, and resources. The platform adopts a multidisciplinary approach that brings together experts from various fields (physiotherapists, social workers, etc.). It can serve as a valuable tool to empower and guide clinicians in their evidence-based telerehabilitation clinical practice, as well as patients and their families in their rehabilitation journey [19].

7.1.3.3 Tele-UPCAT System

Tele-UPCAT application is adapted according to the principles of action observation training (AOT) [20]. The first practical goal is to present a new approach to evaluating bimanual hand functions [20, 21]. The secondary aim is to evaluate the level of participation and quality of life at home and in the community regarding single-handed capacity and bimanual daily activities. The Tele-UPCAT system can be used as a comfortable, reliable, and customizable tool at home for children with cerebral palsy with unilateral involvement and their families [20]. Motor performance evaluation of the system in practice. It consists of the same common objects and toys shown in the videos and is worn on the wrist with two Actigraphs (wGT3X-BT and wActiSleep-BT) used to measure upper extremity activity. It allows quantitative measurements of hand activity, such as force or pressure, during movement observation training with sensory toys embedded in the motor performance module [20].

7.1.3.4 TeleFE

Tele Executive Function is a neuropsychological assessment based on a web platform. It includes four tasks that evaluate inhibition, updating, cognitive flexibility, and planning. This assessment consists of a survey for parents or teachers to obtain information about the child's daily functioning, including executive functions. The test battery evaluates children from 1st grade to 8th grade. Only the planning task from the subparameter of the test can be applied starting from the 3rd grade [22].

7.1.3.4.1 Go/No-Go Task

In this task, the inhibition of responding to the child's capacity to perform alternative actions for the task by suppressing automatic behaviors is evaluated. The task presents a series of geometric shapes on the screen with yellow or blue triangles or circles. Children are instructed to respond to target stimuli while avoiding nontarget stimuli. The mission consists of four blocks with 50 items in each block, 35 Go and 15 No-Go items.

Blocks

The first block consists of yellow figures as Go stimuli and blue figures as No-Go stimuli, regardless of their geometric shape. The second block is applied by reversing the first evaluation. Third block: circles are presented as Go stimuli, and triangles are presented as No-Go stimuli, regardless of color. The fourth block is applied by reversing the third evaluation. Each stimulus is displayed for 500 ms. The stimulus disappears after the child responds or after 500 ms have passed. A neutral screen appears between stimuli. In this task, the mean reaction time to Go stimuli (Go RT), the mean number of accurate responses to No-Go stimuli (No-Go CR), and the mean number of correct responses to Go stimuli (Go CR) are measured. No-Go CR is a measure of the executive function's inhibitory component. Basic processes, Go CR and Go RT are measurements of stimulus elaboration in terms of speed and accuracy, respectively. It measures task commitment and work speed [22].

7.1.3.4.2 Flanker Task

This assessment measures initiative control and cognitive flexibility. Interference control refers to ignoring irrelevant information, while cognitive flexibility involves switching between two rules based on stimulus characteristics. To complete the activity, the youngster must point in the direction of the target arrow on a screen showing five total arrows. The mission comprises three blocks. The first and second blocks contain eight samples and 40 trials, while the third consists of 64 items. The first block is blue, the second is orange, and the third is a combination of blue and orange. Each block contains arrows pointing left or right in 50% of the trials. The screen displays arrows. In the remaining 50%, the arrow in the center points opposite the arrows on the sides. The task involves three blocks. In the first block, the child must indicate the direction of the middle arrow by pressing the letter "R" on the keyboard if the arrow is pointing to the right or "L" if it is pointing to the left. In the second block, the child must indicate the direction of the outer arrows, as in the previous block. The third block involves mixed rules. If the arrows are blue, the rule of the first block is applied. If the arrows are orange, the rule for the second block has been passed. A fixed point appears in the middle of the screen for approximately 600–1200 ms in all blocks. After a white screen lasting 600 ms, the warning is presented for a maximum duration of 1500 ms. To ensure the validity of the response, it must be given at least 200 ms after the stimulus is presented before the stimulus disappears. Finally, the number of correct responses appropriate to the target blocks is recorded and the average time for correct responses is measured. The number of correct responses in the incongruent condition of the central and peripheral target blocks and the average reaction time to correct responses in the incongruent condition of the central and peripheral target blocks are measured. Scores obtained in incongruent conditions are considered a measure of interference control in a single-rule task and a pure measure of cognitive flexibility in a mixed-rule task. In contrast, scores obtained in congruent conditions are considered a measure of multiple stimulus elaboration and task engagement, which are basic processes [22].

7.1.3.4.3 N-Back Task

In this task, it is used to update working memory. The child sees a series of stimuli in the middle of the screen and must press the space bar when the stimulus matches one of the previous stimuli. The task involves colors, shapes, and letters of increasing difficulty. Each condition has two blocks, 1-back and 2-back, respectively, resulting in six blocks. Each block consists of 52 items containing 16 targets. In the N-back task, 1-back and 2-back scores are considered measures of working memory updating at low and high loads, respectively [22].

7.1.3.4.4 Daily Planning Test (DPT)

This task assesses planning ability and ability to select and organize actions to achieve a goal. The child must arrange a schedule for a hypothetical day by defining the order of tasks, completing all tasks by following the fastest route, and adhering to logical and time constraints. The screen displays a map with streets, houses, and shops and a list of 11 activities in random order. The task requires the child to plan various activities that must be completed in different locations and with certain restrictions. The child is shown a list of activities to be planned and is asked to recall them, estimate the time required for each activity, and put them in order. For children aged 11 and over, indicating the time needed to perform each activity is also required. The planning score is represented by the percentage of jobs arranged in the correct order using the map [22].

7.1.3.4.5 Questionnaires for EF Assessment (QUFE)

This assessment tool evaluates a child's executive behavior at home or school. The QUFE comprises 32 items, each rated on a 5-point scale from "not at all true" to "completely true". The parent form of the QUFE considers five executive function components: cognitive self-regulation, behavioural self-regulation, cognitive flexibility, substantive organization, and initiative. The teacher form assesses the student's cognitive and behavioral self-regulation as well as their ability to organize materials. The score is then recorded in its entirety [22].

7.1.3.5 Gross Motor Function-Family Report

Since caregivers can observe the child's skills in the child's living environment, the tools completed observationally by these people have proven valid [23].

Chagas and colleagues developed a family-centered assessment tool—Gross Motor Function-Family. Families reported that it was easy to use, valued the families' knowledge, and suitable for telehealth use. GMF-FR is based on GMFM and is not a new version of GMFM [24].

Differences from GMFM:

1. There are fewer items to measure function.
2. Allows the use of shoes and auxiliary devices/orthoses.
3. Families can report the child's function without needing a therapist using the assessment tool.
4. Photos are added to describe each item.
5. In scale, for each item, binary scoring based on "does" and "does not" is used, which is evaluated according to the criteria.
6. The scale evaluates Performance rather than Capacity as defined in the ICF [25].
7. Eliminates the need for special equipment by allowing furniture to be used in the home environment.
8. GMF-FR can be applied remotely [24].

7.1.3.6 Pediatric Evaluation of Disability Inventory-Computer Adaptive Test (PEDI-CAT)

PEDI-CAT was created to obtain results from the Pediatric Evaluation of Disability Inventory (PEDI) quickly and evaluate children in a wider age group [26–28]. PEDI-CAT evaluates the upper extremity functions of individuals aged 0–21 in daily living activities under four headings. Daily activities are the skills in performing life activities such as eating, dressing, cleaning, using electronic household appliances, and making simple repairs.

The test asks about activities that are more difficult or easier to do, depending on the answers given under these main headings, and this test, which takes an average of 30 min, is answered by the caregivers of the child. Main topics of the PEDI-CAT test:

- Daily activities.
- Ambulation.
- Social/cognitive abilities.
- Responsibility is evaluated [26–28].

References

1. Cheong JL, Burnett AC, Treyvaud K, Spittle AJ. Early environment and long-term outcomes of preterm infants. J Neural Transm. 2020;127:1–8.
2. Spittle A, Orton J, Anderson PJ, Boyd R, Doyle LW. Early developmental intervention programmes provided post hospital discharge to prevent motor and cognitive impairment in preterm infants. Cochrane Database Syst Rev. 2015;2015(11):CD005495.
3. Ustad T, Evensen KAI, Bertoncelli N, Frassoldati R, Ferrari F. Validity of the general movement optimality list in infants born preterm. Pediatr Phys Ther. 2017;29(4):315–20.
4. Martin J, Friel K, Salimi I, Chakrabarty S. Corticospinal development. In: Squire LR, editor. Encyclopedia of neuroscience. Oxford: Academic Press; 2009. p. 302–14.
5. Hadders-Algra M. Early brain damage and the development of motor behavior in children: clues for therapeutic intervention? Neural Plast. 2001;8(1–2):31–49.
6. Cacioppo M, Bouvier S, Bailly R, Houx L, Lempereur M, Mensah-Gourmel J, et al. Emerging health challenges for children with physical disabilities and their parents during the COVID-19 pandemic: the ECHO French survey. Ann Phys Rehabil Med. 2021;64(3):101429.
7. Çelik Ş, Çak E. The effect of the COVID-19 pandemia process on the family. Gevher Nesibe J Med Health Sci. 2021;6(11):43–9.
8. Stein J, Visco CJ, Barbuto S. Rehabilitation medicine response to the COVID-19 pandemic. Am J Phys Med Rehabil. 2020;99(7):573–9.
9. Yağcı HÇ, Bağcıer F. Physical therapy and rehabilitation services after COVID-19. In: Ayhan FF, Demirbağ Kabayel D, editors. COVID19 Pandemisi ve Fiziksel Tıp ve Rehabilitasyon. Ankara: Turkıye Klınıklerı; 2020. p. 94–8.
10. Jeste S, Hyde C, Distefano C, Halladay A, Ray S, Porath M, et al. Changes in access to educational and healthcare services for individuals with intellectual and developmental disabilities during COVID-19 restrictions. J Intellect Disabil Res. 2020;64(11):825–33.
11. Rao PT. A paradigm shift in the delivery of physical therapy services for children with disabilities in the time of the COVID-19 pandemic. Phys Ther. 2021;101(1):pzaa192.

12. Brennan DM, Mawson S, Brownsell S. Telerehabilitation: enabling the remote delivery of healthcare, rehabilitation, and self management. In: Advanced technologies in rehabilitation. IOS Press; 2009. p. 231–48.
13. Dorsey ER, Topol EJ. State of telehealth. N Engl J Med. 2016;375(2):154–61.
14. Peretti A, Amenta F, Tayebati SK, Nittari G, Mahdi SS. Telerehabilitation: re-view of the state-of-the-art and areas of application. JMIR Rehabil Assist Technol. 2017;4(2):e7511.
15. Sarsak HI. Telerehabilitation services: a successful paradigm for occupation-al therapy clinical services. Int Phys Med Rehabil J. 2020;5(2):93–8.
16. Tam JW, Van Son C, Dyck D, Schmitter-Edgecombe M. An educational video program to increase aging services technology awareness among older adults. Patient Educ Couns. 2017;100(8):1564–71.
17. Longo E, De Campos AC, Schiariti V. COVID-19 pandemic: is this a good time for implementation of home programs for children's rehabilitation in low-and middle-income countries? Phys Occup Ther Pediatr. 2020;40(4):361–4.
18. Golomb MR, McDonald BC, Warden SJ, Yonkman J, Saykin AJ, Shirley B, et al. In-home virtual reality videogame telerehabilitation in adolescents with hemiplegic cerebral palsy. Arch Phys Med Rehabil. 2010;91(1):1–8.e1.
19. Ogourtsova T. TelereHUB-CHILD: an online integrated knowledge translation tool to optimize telerehabilitation evidence-based practices for children with disabilities and their families. Front Rehabil Sci. 2023;4:1139432. https://doi.org/10.3389/fresc.2023.1139432.
20. Sgandurra G, Cecchi F, Beani E, Mannari I, Maselli M, Falotico FP, et al. Tele-UPCAT: study protocol of a randomised controlled trial of a home-based Tele-monitored UPper limb Children Action observation Training for participants with unilateral cerebral palsy. BMJ Open. 2018;8(5):e017819.
21. Krumlinde-Sundholm L, Eliasson A-C. Development of the assisting hand assessment: a Rasch-built measure intended for children with unilateral upper limb impairments. Scand J Occup Ther. 2003;10(1):16–26.
22. Rivella C, Ruffini C, Bombonato C, Capodieci A, Frascari A, Marzocchi GM, et al. TeleFE: a new tool for the tele-assessment of executive functions in children. Appl Sci. 2023;13(3):1728.
23. Coster W, Law M, Bedell G, Khetani M, Cousins M, Teplicky R. Development of the participation and environment measure for children and youth: conceptual basis. Disabil Rehabil. 2012;34(3):238–46.
24. Chagas PS, Rosenbaum P, Wright FV, Pritchard L, Wright M, Martins Toledo A, et al. Development of the Gross Motor Function Family Report (GMF-FR) for children with cerebral palsy. Physiother Can. 2023;75(1):83–91.
25. World Health Organization. International classification of functioning, disability, and health: children & youth version: ICF-CY. World Health Organization; 2007.
26. Haley SM, Coster W, Ludlow LH, Haltiwanger JT, Andrellos PJ. Pediatric evaluation of disability inventory (PEDI). Health and Disability Research Institute Boston University; 1992.
27. Ziviani J, Ottenbacher KJ, Shephard K, Foreman S, Astbury W, Ireland P. Concurrent validity of the functional independence measure for children (WeeF-IM (™)) and the pediatric evaluation of disabilities inventory in children with developmental disabilities and acquired brain injuries. Phys Occup Ther Pediatr. 2002;21(2–3):91–101.
28. Haley SM, Coster WJ, Dumas HM, Fragala-Pinkham MA, Kramer J, Ni P, et al. Accuracy and precision of the Pediatric Evaluation of Disability Inventory computer-adaptive tests (PEDI-CAT). Dev Med Child Neurol. 2011;53(12):1100–6.

8 Telerehabilitation Methods in Pediatric Rehabilitation

Nejla Uzun

8.1 Introduction

Families of children with complex health needs who have difficulty accessing specialist services due to problems in geography and healthcare organizations may not be able to access adequate healthcare because it is more time-consuming, costly, and distressing. This insufficient access can lead to inadequate healthcare for children [1].

Technology is an important tool that enables patients to access healthcare services more easily and at less cost [1, 2]. Telehealth is a broad concept for interventions that include technologies that allow remote data exchange between patients and healthcare professionals to support the management and diagnosis of health conditions. The use of technologies such as Internet services, telephone, videoconferencing, e-mail, and self-monitoring equipment allows many services to be provided remotely, such as remote monitoring of patients [2]. At the same time, telehealth has been shown in the literature to be a useful method for improving the skills of the local health workforce [3].

Telerehabilitation is considered a subfield of telehealth and aims to provide remote control or rehabilitation monitoring using telecommunication and information technologies [4, 5]. Telerehabilitation aims to expand rehabilitation opportunities using computer-aided systems, offer health services in rural areas, improve the quality of life, eliminate close contact between the clinician and the patient in cases where it is not possible or risky to go to rehabilitation centers during epidemic periods, reduce medical costs and save time and resources in health services [4–7]. Telerehabilitation content is similar to rehabilitation services provided face-to-face in normal times, with individual interviews, patient evaluations, rehabilitation goals,

N. Uzun (✉)
Istanbul Galata University, İstanbul, Turkey
e-mail: nejla.uzun@galata.edu.tr

F. Özden et al. (eds.), *Telerehabilitation*, TELe-Health,
https://doi.org/10.1007/978-3-031-69080-8_8

and individual exercise programs [8]. It allows physiotherapists to continue examining the musculoskeletal system, distance education with consultation, physical evaluation, planning the exercise program required for the patient, and monitoring the patient's progress by providing continuous feedback [9].

Although healthcare professionals have used telerehabilitation for a long time, it has received renewed attention with the COVID-19 pandemic. Many health professionals worldwide and in our country have started to use online consultancy and evaluation methods and have increased their use [9].

Telemedicine has been the main approach to delivering pediatric healthcare during the COVID-19 pandemic when it is accessible, available, and appropriate to address the present problem. Telerehabilitation has increased in pediatric patients to comply with social distancing rules and maintain access to the established care and treatment plan [10]. It has been stated that including modern information and communication technologies, such as telerehabilitation, in home-based rehabilitation programs for patients with neurological problems provides advantages in terms of flexible programming, more comprehensive rehabilitation practices, personalized programs, and easy applicability [11].

8.1.1 Advantages of Pediatric Telerehabilitation

- This model's biggest advantage is reducing the treatment gap by providing door-to-door healthcare services to needy child patients, especially those in remote areas.
- It reduces the need for patients to go to a rehabilitation center to receive services and reduces costs for both healthcare providers and patients.
- It minimizes the disadvantages of situations where social distance must be maintained.
- Family education ensures that the family actively participates in the treatment [12].

8.1.2 Disadvantages

- It can eliminate the therapeutic effects of touch in treatment [12].
- There are concerns about ensuring patient confidentiality.

8.1.3 Difficulties

- The patient may encounter equipment obstructions. The efficiency of the treatment may decrease as a result of encountering equipment obstacles [13].
- There may be a lack of technological knowledge and equipment between the patient and the healthcare unit [14].
- There may be economic constraints [15].
- There may be some problems in user usage [16].

8.2 Cerebral Palsy

Cerebral Palsy (CP) is a disease that causes movement disorders in two to three out of every thousand live births. There are various categories of cerebral palsy, including spasticity (the most common), ataxia, dyskinesia, or a mixed type [17]. Individuals with CP also experience motor learning difficulties and basic limitations in the postural control of dynamic and static tasks such as walking, standing, and sitting. This clinical picture may also include sensory, cognition, communication, and perception—behavioral disorders, seizures, vision and hearing disorders, hip dislocation, scoliosis, and communication difficulties.

Action Observation Therapy (AOT) is a neurorehabilitation-based treatment approach that supports central nervous system restoration by imitating the same movements after monitoring movements, using the neurophysiological mechanism known as the mirror mechanism [18]. Mirror therapy is thought to have a similar neurophysiology to the Action Observation Therapy approach in that it activates the mirror neuron system. However, in mirror therapy, the person's unaffected extremity is used for treatment, while in AOT, the activities in the relevant extremity of another person are watched live or via video [19]. AOT is a low-cost approach that can be easily adapted to the patient population and specific needs of the patients. For this reason, it has been used frequently in recent years, especially in pediatric telerehabilitation [20–23].

In the study conducted by Molinaro et al., ten children with CP, aged between 5 and 12, were followed at home with the AOT program under the supervision of a child neurologist. Video clips with a total duration of 9–12 min were selected from actions that children are familiar with, such as using a pencil and playing with Lego. Each rehabilitation session lasted approximately half an hour, as each action was devoted to observing for 9–12 min and performing the observed actions for 6–8 min. After 2 months of follow-up, as a result of the Melbourne Assessment of Unilateral Upper Limb Function Scale and the Assisting Hand Assessment, it was determined that the children's upper extremity functionality increased, and it was stated that this treatment method was an approach that could be integrated with telerehabilitation [21].

Beani et al. aimed to evaluate the feasibility of a home-based rehabilitation method called "Tele-monitored UPper Limb Children Action Observation Training" (Tele-UPCAT) in pediatric CP patients. In the study of 29 children diagnosed with unilateral CP, a program based on AOT principles was applied in the Tele-UPCAT system. The child watched a video of daily activities targeting the functionality of the upper extremity, such as holding an object and using a pencil. Each activity was shot from different angles and in subdivided stages (such as taking the candy from the table, bringing it closer to the mouth, and giving it back to the therapist). Each activity's video clip lasted 9–12 min, consisting of 3-min periods. Then, the child performed the activity he watched in the video with the "Actigraph" device on his wrist. The program was conducted under the caregiver's supervision, at home on the computer, for 3 weeks, with each session lasting approximately 45 min so that the child could perform the activity with fewer errors. The results emphasized the feasibility of home-based AOT in children and adolescents diagnosed with unilateral CP [22].

Beanie et al. implemented a home program based on AOT principles on the Tele-UPCAT platform for 30 children diagnosed with unilateral CP. This study supports the effectiveness of AOT-based home training in improving upper extremity skills [24].

In their study, Rodríguez-Costa et al. aimed to evaluate whether a telecare intervention consisting of Action Observation Therapy with a family-centered approach improves functionality in children and adolescents with CP. Seven girls with CP, aged between 6 and 17, participated in this case series study, which lasted 12 weeks: A 6-week tele-care program consisting of six sessions and a follow-up period of 6 weeks. This study applied six sessions of AOT with the family center approach. Statistically, significant improvements in gross motor function and clinical changes in balance, walking speed, and endurance were obtained in the short term. There have also been substantial improvements in balance and endurance in the long term [18].

Nuara et al. aimed to evaluate the feasibility and effectiveness of a home-based AOT platform that promotes child-child interaction to improve hand motor function in unilateral CP. In the study, 20 children with unilateral CP were administered 20 sessions in which they had to observe and then imitate a magician performing magic tricks that required manual dexterity. This was followed by an interactive child-to-child session in which two children interacted via video link while repeating the same exercises. As a result of this study, it was emphasized that traditional AOT is effective as a telerehabilitation method [22].

Children and adolescents accept low-cost virtual reality exercise games and technological tools for the ludic, motivating, and engaging features that make them easy to incorporate into telerehabilitation [25, 26]. Golomb et al. aimed to investigate the effectiveness of In-Home Virtual Reality Video Game Handheld Telerehabilitation Intervention in a 15-year-old adolescent with hemiplegic cerebral palsy. The telerehabilitation system included a 5DT 5 Ultra Glove, a 26-inch high-definition TV, a keyboard, and a PlayStation 3 game console programmed with custom rehabilitation games. Hand function was measured using grip strength and the Jebsen hand function test. A total of 14 months after the end of the intervention, repeat assessment demonstrated increased hand function and preservation of forearm bone health [27].

Gatica-Rojas et al. aimed to determine the feasibility and effectiveness of a rehabilitation program using low-cost virtual reality, aiming to improve postural control in children with CP (spastic hemiplegia). The program, which will last 6 weeks and consist of three 25-min sessions per week, was created, and low-cost virtual reality therapy was applied through face-to-face and telerehabilitation methods using the Nintendo Wii balance board. The results of this study emphasized that low-cost virtual reality would improve postural control, help support remote access to rehabilitation services, and provide higher-intensity interventions compared to standard interventions [25].

Move-it-to-Improve-It (Mitii™) is another method used in the rehabilitation of children diagnosed with CP. Mitii™ is a web-based therapy program comprising upper extremity, cognitive, visual perception, and physical activity training. This system can be used at home with a computer and computer camera. It can detect movements with bands attached to the hand, knee, or head [28, 29]. Mitii web-based rehabilitation system offers a cost-effective alternative to improve upper limb function for children with mild to moderate upper limb CP when conventional treatment is unavailable [30].

The home program is defined as "therapeutic activities carried out by the child at home with the help of parents to achieve health-related goals." It is used as a guide and support in many physiotherapy methods. The main goal of the home program is to increase the activity level of children with CP, to prevent secondary problems that can be seen in the long term, and to ensure that acquired skills are used in daily life. Therefore, it is an important approach for pediatric physiotherapists [31].

Sel et al. aimed to compare motor function, activity, and participation between preschool children with CP receiving routine physiotherapy and rehabilitation and children receiving a "Telerehabilitation-Based Structured Home Program" in addition to routine physiotherapy and rehabilitation. A total of 43 children with CP were included in the study, 23 in the study group and 20 in the control group. The telerehabilitation-based Structured Home Program consisted of phases of telerehabilitation and structured home program, and 56 h of therapy were applied at home by the children's parents. Each session of TR lasted 1 h, and the structured home program training was designed specifically for each child. The physiotherapist followed the families through online meetings and regular meetings every week. As a result of the study comparing the control group that received only ordinary care in preschool children with CP and the study group in which the Telerehabilitation-Based Structured Home Program was applied in addition to the usual care, it was emphasized that the Telerehabilitation-Based Structured Home Program could be an effective method for preschool children with CP [31].

Ortega-Martínez et al. applied home-based mirror therapy, including therapist coaching, to six children aged 8–12 years old with a diagnosis of Unilateral Spastic Cerebral Palsy for 30 min a day, 5 days a week, for 5 weeks. While performing the therapy, children were asked to place the affected upper extremity in a Mirror Box in their sagittal plane. All exercises are designed to be performed by the children themselves; parents, on the other hand, are concerned with maintaining the supervision and concentration of their children. The results highlighted that the home-based Mirror Therapy program, where the therapist is involved as a coach throughout the program, is a safe, cost-effective, and feasible therapy for children with CP [32].

Surana et al. compared children who received Lower Extremity Intensive Functional Training (LIFT) with those who received Home-Based Hand-Arm Bimanual Intensive Therapy (H-HABIT). Children diagnosed with unilateral CP with levels I-II according to the Gross Motor Function Classification System (GMFCS) were included in the study. The exercises of both groups were composed of functional exercises that included daily living activities. LIFT was applied to one group for 90 h, and H-HABIT at an equal dose (2 h a day, 5 days a week, for

9 weeks) was applied to the other group. The 2-h training is divided into two periods of 1 h or four periods of 30 min during the day. The participants were monitored 1 day a week, 1 h a day, using telerehabilitation. How the participants did their exercises was monitored, and changes were made to the program when necessary. As a result of the training, it was concluded that LIFT training provided positive development in ambulation distance and general walking ability [33].

Telerehabilitation has significant effectiveness in improving functions (gait capacity and performance, occupational performance, manual dexterity, bimanual hand function, and lower extremity function) in children with Unilateral CP whose age range is between 2 and 18 years, with GMFCS levels I and II, and MACS levels I, II, and III. However, children with GMFCS levels III, IV, and V and MACS levels IV and V were omitted as there was no evidence to support this hypothesis [34].

8.3 Duchenne Muscular Dystrophy and Becker Muscular Dystrophy

Duchenne muscular dystrophy (DMD) and Becker muscular dystrophy (BMD) are rare neuromuscular diseases caused by a mutation in the dystrophin-producing gene [35]. The worldwide prevalence of BMD is approximately 1 in 3500 male individuals and 0.5 in 10,000 male individuals for DMD [36]. In the clinical course of DMD, patients develop progressive loss of motor function, gait abnormalities, progressive respiratory failure, and cardiomyopathy [37]. BMD is clinically similar to DMD, where weakness and weakness of mostly proximally located muscles are more common. However, BMD has a slower and milder course compared to DMD. Walking difficulties usually begin after the age of 16. International guidelines state that regular physical activity and occupational and speech therapies are necessary for DMD patients in home, school, and outpatient settings [38].

Telerehabilitation in patients with DMD can be performed using video techniques, with training of caregivers, during the pandemic period when patients discontinue institutional physical therapy due to national recommendations on social isolation and in cases where there is limited participation in institutional rehabilitation [39]. VR in physiotherapy and rehabilitation programs for children can provide personalized treatment by allowing us to increase sensory feedback, attention, and motivation and integrate the child's preferences into the intervention program [35].

Baeza-Barragán et al. investigated the effectiveness of a 5-week Virtual Reality-based Telerehabilitation Program in their study with 12 children diagnosed with DMD and BMD. The participants were first subjected to the control condition, where they were first applied to a conventional physical therapy program without using VR glasses, and then functional tests were performed. Then, an intervention condition consisting of ten 30-min sessions was applied, including self-stretching, aerobic exercise, yoga, mindfulness, breathing and relaxation, and training with VR glasses. A 6-minute walk test, North Star Ambulatory Assessment, timed up and go test, and Motor Function Measure were used to evaluate the participants. No difference was found between conventional and telerehabilitation treatments in the results, and it was emphasized that telerehabilitation helped preserve motor function in children with DMD and BMD [35].

In a study evaluating the feasibility of pulmonary rehabilitation practiced via telerehabilitation in DMD patients, children and their families were taught positive inspiratory and expiratory pressure and glossopharyngeal breathing during an online conference. It is recommended to do these exercises every day, three times a day, without the support of a physiotherapist. Although the study concluded that it is possible to implement respiratory telerehabilitation, which includes the feedback of families and the help of caregivers, the authors stated that there is little interest in digital rehabilitation among children's caregivers in Poland [40].

8.4 Myelomeningocele

Myelomeningocele (MMC) is a congenital disease in which the neural tube does not close completely and is associated with varying degrees of motor and sensory loss depending on the level of the lesion, as well as neurogenic bowel-bladder problems, hydrocephalus, and Arnold Chiari malformation [41]. Because children and adults with MMC often have long-term physical and cognitive disabilities and developmental delays that affect daily functioning, they need assistance with self-care activities and ambulation. Physiotherapy and rehabilitation approaches should be applied regularly to increase muscle strength and tone of patients diagnosed with MMC, improve sitting and walking functions, and protect the child's development and functionality by preventing contractures [42].

In a study examining the effectiveness and feasibility of occupational-based telerehabilitation in adolescents diagnosed with myelomeningocele, the "Cognitive Orientation to Daily Occupational Performance" (CO-OP) program was carried out through a teleconferencing application (Skype™) using the participants' tablet or home computer [43]. The CO-OP approach is situated within a learning paradigm and uses cognitive strategies to facilitate skill acquisition at the ICF activity rather than at the level of structure and function and draws on motor learning principles to help children explore. The main objectives of CO-OP are skill acquisition, learning a global problem-solving strategy, and identification of domain-specific strategies [44]. During these sessions, which lasted 30–60 min for 10–12 weeks, the patient's goals were determined, and the program was followed. If the program could not be realized, objectives, performance, plans, and strategies were discussed in the sessions. The evaluation was made before, after, and 3 months after the end of the application, and Canadian Occupational Performance Measure, Pediatric Functional Independence Measure, and Pediatric Quality of Life Inventory were used in the evaluation. After ten sessions, significant gains were achieved in the patient's goals, improvement in daily living activities was observed, and it was concluded that this approach positively affected participation and independence in myelomeningocele patients [43].

8.5 Arthrogryposis Multiplex Congenita

Arthrogryposis multiplex congenita (AMC) is a disease that causes joint contractures in at least two body regions, a decrease in muscle mass and consequent compensations, pain, activity and participation restrictions, and limitation in daily living activities. AMC, which requires specialized multidisciplinary care, is provided in large urban areas that are not easily accessible to many people with AMC. Therefore, developing approaches that allow remote management of the patient's clinical problems may benefit this population [45]. Due to the worldwide COVID-19 pandemic, there has been increased interest in various digital application opportunities, such as telerehabilitation, used to provide remote patient assessments and interventions [46]. Telerehabilitation offers greater accessibility, lower costs, and less patient travel time [47].

In the study of youth with AMC aged 8–21 years, a remote multidisciplinary teleassessment, including active ROM assessment, was conducted by a physical therapist and an occupational therapist before starting the telerehabilitation intervention and at the end of the 12-week intervention. All teleassessments were performed using the Zoom Pro videoconferencing system. A virtual goniometer was used to measure the ROM of the upper and lower extremities of youth with AMC based on screenshots. The study results show that virtual goniometry is repeatable and reproducible for the ROM of most joints [45].

In a study evaluating the effectiveness of home-based exercise, physical activity level, functional level, and pain were assessed using the "Physical Activity Questionnaire for Adolescents," "Pediatrics Outcomes Data Collection Instrument," and "Adolescent Pediatric Pain Tool" scales before and after a 12-week individual program implementation. Before the program, individual goals were determined with the "Goal Attainment Scale." The joint range of motion was evaluated with a virtual goniometer in the first telerehabilitation session. As a result of the study, positive improvements were detected in physical activity level, functional level, pain, and goal-oriented work performance [47].

8.6 Autism Spectrum Disorder

Autism spectrum disorder (ASD) is a pervasive developmental disorder characterized by difficulties with behavior and speech, such as repetitive behaviors, lack of social abilities, communication disorders, and activity and interest disorders with limitations [48]. In addition to social interaction, communication, and behavioral disorders, the motor skills of autistic patients often do not develop [49]. Autistic patients generally have low physical activity levels due to their social and behavioral deficits. It has been shown in many studies that physical activity improves the physical and mental health of autistic patients in basic symptoms and reduces the risk of some chronic diseases such as obesity [50]. Telerehabilitation for children diagnosed with autism offers the opportunity to learn with a robot at school or clinic and at home. Information about robot-based telerehabilitation applications in these patients was reported for the first time in 2010 [51].

Almeida et al. aimed to evaluate telerehabilitation's feasibility, pleasure, and potential impact using the VR platform called "MoveHero." In the study, which evaluated 22 families of individuals with ASD and 22 individuals without ASD matched to the experimental group in terms of age and gender, a platform called MoveHero, which is available for free in Portuguese and English, was used. The MoveHero platform, where the participant is positioned in front of a computer and when the game begins, the webcam captures the participant's movements so that a representation of the player appears as an avatar on the computer screen, also includes a musical beat to increase engagement. The parents of the participants were contacted via phone and video call. During the video call, parents and guardians were given all instructions on how to do the game and how to perform the tasks, and individuals with ASD were given researcher-led telerehabilitation at home. The parents of the participants were contacted via video call. During the video call, parents and guardians were given all instructions on how to perform the tasks, and parents and guardians were asked to help individuals with ASD carry out telerehabilitation sessions at home under the leadership of the researcher. The Childhood Autism Rating Scale, Brunel Mood Scale, Enjoyment Scale, and Rating of Perceived Exertion-CR10 were used in the assessment. As a result of the study, it was emphasized that the intervention was safe and applicable for participating children with autism. It was stated that all participants performed better in repeated trials, and most participants (~60%) enjoyed the games at a very high level [52].

Parsons et al. randomly divided 59 children with ASD between the ages of 2 and 6 into two groups. Therapy Outcomes by You (TOBY), an iPad application and intervention tool developed by a team of Western Australian computer scientists, psychologists, and speech pathologists, was used in the study. TOBY practice includes high-intensity interventions to meet the needs of individual children using behavioral, educational, and developmental approaches focusing on four major skill areas (visual motor, imitation, language, and social). This study suggested that, compared to therapy as usual, TOBY treatment provided benefits in expressive language for children with ASD living in regional areas of Western Australia. Additionally, significant gains were observed from the intervention in receptive and pragmatic language and social skills [53].

A feasibility study of parent training was conducted with children aged 3–8 years with ASD and disruptive behavior living in rural areas. The RUBI-PT program, which includes 11 core sessions, up to two additional sessions, and three telephone support sessions, was carried out by four trained therapists for 6 months. The Behavioral Interventions Research Unit (RUBI) Autism Network is a structured Parent Training (PT) program that targets common behavioral problems in children with ASD, such as tantrums, noncompliance, and aggression. Results from this pilot trial support the feasibility and preliminary effectiveness of the 24-week RUBI parent training program for children with autism and disruptive behavior when delivered via telehealth [54].

Agdassi et al. aimed to investigate the effect of "Sports, Play and Active Recreation for Kids" (SPARK), a family-centered motor program to develop gross motor skills in children diagnosed with high-functioning ASD. This program includes rope skipping, walking, running, jumping, warm-up, and cool-down. The sessions were taught to the family over the phone, and the families applied the program to their children 3 days a week for 8 weeks, each lasting 45 min. The results showed that family-based telerehabilitation significantly improved gross motor skills in children diagnosed with high-functioning ASD and could be an alternative approach for children and families who cannot reach rehabilitation centers [55].

Su et al. aimed to compare the acceptability, feasibility, accuracy, and effectiveness of telehealth, face-to-face standard care, and SP intervention to improve fine motor and social communication skills in children with autism spectrum disorder. Sitting play interventions were applied to 15 children with ASD (Face-to-face Subgroup ($n = 7$), Tele-health Subgroup ($n = 8$)) twice a week for 8 weeks. Seated play group includes standard care, supplemental instruction, and special education-based activities, including greetings and farewells, fine motor games, reading storybooks, building activities using Play-Doh and Legos, and arts and crafts activities. As a result of the study, it was emphasized that there were similar improvements in fine motor performance and social communication in children with ASD after telehealth and face-to-face interventions and that both intervention methods were considered satisfactory, appropriate, useful, and possible for parents to implement with their children [56].

8.7 Acute Lymphoblastic Leukemia

Acute Lymphoblastic Leukemia (ALL) is the most common pediatric hematological malignancy. ALL and its treatment negatively affect bone mineral balance, causing late musculoskeletal side effects. With the increase in the survival rate in childhood cancers, the frequency of late side effects increases, and an inactive lifestyle exacerbates these side effects. A telerehabilitation program is recommended to strengthen the muscle-bone complex and minimize late-term side effects [57].

Lambert et al. aimed to evaluate the feasibility of a supervised telehealth home exercise intervention for early survivors of bone marrow-related hematological malignancies. The study included 40 potential home-based physical activity interventions, supervised by a kinesiologist via a telehealth Internet platform, with monthly progression. The study showed that the approach was applicable and effective in the musculoskeletal system [58].

A home-based physical activity program was implemented in the study, in which children who had completed ALL treatments were included in a group treatment program using the telerehabilitation method. Before the program, the physiotherapist went to the children's homes and installed the materials to help the families with technology, room layout, and parameters. Children were supervised for 16 weeks by a physiotherapist via an online platform. The home-based physical activity program is designed to be progressive, increasing in duration or frequency each month (2–3 days/week, 35–45 min/day). Exercises were adapted or changed in each session according to the pain level of the participants. In the interviews held after the treatment program, both children and their parents expressed that they were very satisfied with the program, and they also stated that they would recommend this program to other families in a similar situation [57].

References

1. Edirippulige S, Reyno J, Armfield NR, Bambling M, Lloyd O, McNevin E. Availability, spatial accessibility, utilisation and the role of telehealth for multi-disciplinary paediatric cerebral palsy services in Queensland. J Telemed Telecare. 2016;22(7):391–6.
2. Kayyali R, Hesso I, Mahdi A, Hamzat O, Adu A, Nabhani Gebara S. Telehealth: misconceptions and experiences of healthcare professionals in England. Int J Pharm Pract. 2017;25(3):203–9.
3. Moffatt JJ, Eley DS. The reported benefits of telehealth for rural Australians. Aust Health Rev. 2010;34:276–81.
4. Rogante M, Grigioni M, Cordella D, Giacomozzi C. Ten years of telerehabilitation: a literature overview of technologies and clinical applications. NeuroRehabilitation. 2010;27(4):287–304.
5. Brienza DM, McCue M. Introduction to telerehabilitation. In: Telerehabilitation. London: Springer; 2013. p. 1–11.
6. Kairy D, Lehoux P, Vincent C, Visintin M. A systematic review of clinical outcomes, clinical process, healthcare utilization and costs associated with telerehabilitation. Disabil Rehabil. 2009;31(6):427–47.
7. Kahraman T. Koronavirüs hastalığı (COVID-19) pandemisi ve telerehabilitasyon. İzmir Katip Çelebi Üniversitesi Sağlık Bilimleri Fakültesi Dergisi. 2020;5(2):87–92.
8. Purssell E, Gould D, Chudleigh J. Impact of isolation on hospitalised patients who are infectious: systematic review with meta-analysis. BMJ Open. 2020;10(2):e030371.
9. Smith AC, Thomas E, et al. Telehealth for global emergencies: implications for coronavirus disease 2019 (COVID-19). J Telemed Telecare. 2020;26(5):309–13.
10. Badawy SM, Radovic A. Digital approaches to remote pediatric health care delivery during the COVID-19 pandemic: existing evidence and a call for further research. JMIR Pediatr Parent. 2020;3(1):e20049.
11. Çelikel R, Ramazanoglu E, Talu B. The effect of motor learning-based telerehabilitation on quality of life of children with cerebral palsy during the COVID-19 pandemic. Arch Pediatr. 2023;30(6):383–8.
12. Mishra V. Factors affecting the adoption of telemedicine during COVID-19. Indian J Public Health. 2020;64(Suppl):S234–6.
13. Howard IM, Kaufman MS. Telehealth applications for outpatients with neuromuscular or musculoskeletal disorders. Muscle Nerve. 2018;58(4):475–85.
14. Ferre CL, Brandão M, Surana B, Dew AP, Moreau NG, Gordon AM. Caregiver-directed home-based intensive bimanual training in young children with unilateral spastic cerebral palsy: a randomized trial. Dev Med Child Neurol. 2017;59(5):497–504.
15. Salawu A, Green A, Crooks MG, Brixey N, Ross DH, Sivan M. A proposal for multidisciplinary tele-rehabilitation in the assessment and rehabilitation of COVID-19 survivors. Int J Environ Res Public Health. 2020;17(13):4890.
16. Fiani B, Siddiqi I, Lee SC, Dhillon L. Telerehabilitation: development, application, and need for increased usage in the COVID-19 era for patients with spinal pathology. Cureus. 2020;12(9):e10563.
17. Gonzalez NA, Sanivarapu RR, Osman U, Kumar AL, Sadagopan A, Mahmoud A, et al. Physical therapy interventions in children with cerebral palsy: a systematic review. Cureus. 2023;15(8):e43846.

18. Rodríguez-Costa I, Abuín-Porras V, Terán-García P, Férez-Sopeña A, Calvo-Fuente V, Soto-Vidal C, Pacheco-da-Costa S. Effectiveness of a telecare physical therapy program in improving functionality in children and adolescents with cerebral palsy: a cases study. Children. 2023;10(4):663.
19. Buccino G. Action observation treatment: a novel tool in neurorehabilitation. Philos Trans R Soc Lond B Biol Sci. 2014;369(1644):20130185.
20. Erturan S, Burak M, Elbasan B. Improving upper extremity functionality in children with unilateral cerebral palsy with action observation therapy. Igusabder. 2022;18:1052–69.
21. Molinaro A, Micheletti S, Pagani F, et al. Action observation treatment in a tele-rehabilitation setting: a pilot study in children with cerebral palsy. Disabil Rehabil. 2020;44(7):1107–12.
22. Beani E, Menici V, Ferrari A, Cioni G, Sgandurra G. Feasibility of a home-based action observation training for children with unilateral cerebral palsy: an explorative study. Front Neurol. 2020;11:16.
23. Nuara A, Avanzini P, Rizzolatti G, Fabbri-Destro M. Efficacy of a home-based platform for child-to-child interaction on hand motor function in unilateral cerebral palsy. Dev Med Child Neurol. 2019;61(11):1314–22.
24. Beani E, Menici V, Sicola E, Ferrari A, Feys H, Klingels K, et al. Effectiveness of the home-based training program tele-UPCAT (tele-monitored upper limb children action observation training) in unilateral cerebral palsy: a randomized controlled trial. Eur J Phys Rehabil Med. 2023;59(5):554–63.
25. Gatica-Rojas V, Cartes-Velásquez R, Soto-Poblete A, Lizama LEC. Postural control telerehabilitation with a low-cost virtual reality protocol for children with cerebral palsy: protocol for a clinical trial. PLoS One. 2023;18(8):e0268163.
26. Westby A, Nissly T, Gieseker R, Timmins K, Justesen K. Achieving equity in telehealth: "centering at the margins" in access, provision, and reimbursement. J Am Board Fam Med. 2021;34(Suppl):29–32.
27. Golomb MR, Warden SJ, Fess E, Rabin B, Yonkman J, Shirley B, Burdea GC. Maintained hand function and forearm bone health 14 months after an in-home virtual-reality videogame hand telerehabilitation intervention in an adolescent with hemiplegic cerebral palsy. J Child Neurol. 2011;26(3):389–93.
28. Piovesana AM, Ross S, Lloyd O, et al. Randomized controlled trial of a web-based multimodal therapy program for executive functioning in children and adolescents with unilateral cerebral palsy. Disabil Rehabil. 2017;39(20):2021–8.
29. Boyd RN, Baque E, Piovesana A, Ross S, Ziviani J, Sakzewski L, et al. Mitii™ ABI: study protocol of a randomised controlled trial of a web-based multi-modal training program for children and adolescents with an Acquired Brain Injury (ABI). BMC Neurol. 2015;15:1–29.
30. Comans T, Mihala G, Sakzewski L, Boyd RN, Scuffham P. The cost-effectiveness of a web-based multimodal therapy for unilateral cerebral palsy: the Mitii randomized controlled trial. Dev Med Child Neurol. 2017;59(7):756–61.
31. Sel SA, Günel MK, Erdem S, Tunçdemir M. Effects of telerehabilitation-based structured home program on activity, participation and goal achievement in preschool children with cerebral palsy: a triple-blinded randomized controlled trial. Children. 2023;10(3):424.
32. Ortega-Martínez A, Palomo-Carrión R, Varela-Ferro C, Bagur-Calafat MC. Feasibility of a home-based mirror therapy program in children with unilateral spastic cerebral palsy. Healthcare. 2023;11(12):1797.
33. Surana BK, Ferre CL, Dew AP, Brandao M, Gordon AM, Moreau NG. Effectiveness of Lower-Extremity Functional Training (LIFT) in young children with unilateral spastic cerebral palsy: a randomized controlled trial. Neurorehabil Neural Repair. 2019;33(10):862–72.
34. Tamboosi ME, Al-Khathami SS, El-Shamy SM. The effectiveness of tele-rehabilitation on improvement of daily living activities in children with cerebral palsy: narrative review. BFPT. 2021;26(1):1–12.
35. Baeza-Barragán MR, Labajos Manzanares MT, Amaya-Álvarez MC, Morales Vega F, Rodriguez Ruiz J, Martín-Valero R. Effectiveness of a 5-week virtual reality telerehabilitation

program for children with Duchenne and Becker muscular dystrophy: prospective quasi-experimental study. JMIR Serious Games. 2023;11:e48022.
36. Nascimento Osorio A, Medina Cantillo J, Camacho Salas A, Madruga Garrido M, Vilchez Padilla JJ. Consensus on the diagnosis, treatment and follow-up of patients with Duchenne muscular dystrophy. Neurología. 2019;34(7):469–81.
37. Mosqueira M, Zeiger U, Förderer M, Brinkmeier H, Fink RH. Cardiac and respiratory dysfunction in Duchenne muscular dystrophy and the role of second messengers. Med Res Rev. 2013;33(5):1174–213.
38. Birnkrant DJ, Bushby K, Bann CM, et al. Diagnosis and management of Duchenne muscular dystrophy, part 1: diagnosis, and neuromuscular, rehabilitation, endocrine, and gastrointestinal and nutritionalmanagement. Lancet Neurol. 2018;17(3):251–67.
39. Sobierajska-Rek A, Mański Ł, Jabłońska-Brudło J, Śledzińska K, Ucińska A, Wierzba J. Establishing a telerehabilitation program for patients with Duchenne muscular dystrophy in the COVID-19 pandemic. Wien Klin Wochenschr. 2021;133(7–8):344–50.
40. Sobierajska-Rek A, Mański Ł, Jabłońska-Brudło J, Śledzińska K, Wasilewska E, Szalewska D. Respiratory telerehabilitation of boys and young men with Duchenne muscular dystrophy in the COVID-19 pandemic. Int J Environ Res Public Health. 2021;18(12):6179.
41. Komolafe EO, Onyia CU, Ogunbameru IO, et al. The pattern, peculiarities, and management challenges of spina bifida in a teaching hospital in Southwest Nigeria. Childs Nerv Syst. 2018;34(2):311–9.
42. Baym CL, Hedgecock JB, Rapport MJK. Functional mobility improved after intensive progressive resistance exercise in an adolescent with spina bifida. Pediatr Phys Ther. 2018;30(2):1–7.
43. Steinhart S, Raz-Silbiger S, Beeri M, Gilboa Y. Occupation based telerehabilitation intervention for adolescents with myelomeningocele: a pilot study. Phys Occup Ther Pediatr. 2020;41(2):176–91.
44. Cameron D, Craig T, Edwards B, Missiuna C, Schwellnus H, Polatajko HJ. Cognitive orientation to daily occupational performance (CO-OP): a new approach for children with cerebral palsy. Phys Occup Ther Pediatr. 2017;37(2):183–98.
45. Gagnon M, Merlo GM, Dahan-Oliel N, Veilleux LN. Measurement repeatability and reproducibility of virtual goniometry of a set of acquired images in youths with arthrogryposis multiplex congenita. J Musculoskelet Neuronal Interact. 2023;23(2):175.
46. Turolla A, Rossettini G, Viceconti A, Palese A, Geri T. Musculoskeletal physical therapy during the COVID-19 pandemic: is telerehabilitation the answer? Phys Ther. 2020;100(8):1260–4.
47. Gagnon M, Marino Merlo G, Yap R, Collins J, Elfassy C, Sawatzky B, et al. Using telerehabilitation to deliver a home exercise program to youth with arthrogryposis: single cohort pilot study. J Med Internet Res. 2021;23(7):e27064.
48. Xue SY. A study on how sports skills influence children with autism. Mod Commun. 2019;13:209–10.
49. Fournier KA, Hass CJ, Naik SK, Lodha N, Cauraugh JH. Motor coordination in autism spectrum disorders: a synthesis and meta-analysis. J Autism Dev Disord. 2010;40:1227–40.
50. Huang J, Du C, Liu J, Tan G. Meta-analysis on intervention effects of physical activities on children and adolescents with autism. Int J Environ Res Public Health. 2020;17(6):1950.
51. Gillesen J, Boere S, Barakova E. WikiTherapist. In: Proceedings of the 28th annual European conference on cognitive ergonomics, New York; 2010.
52. Almeida AFSD, Silva TDD, Moraes ÍAPD, Menezes LDCD, Dias ED, Araújo LVD, et al. Virtual reality as a telerehabilitation strategy for people with autism spectrum disorder during the COVID-19 quarantine scenario: physical activity, motor performance and enjoyment. Disabil Rehabil Assist Technol. 2024;19(5):2046–56.
53. Parsons D, Cordier R, Lee H, Falkmer T, Vaz S. A randomised controlled trial of an information communication technology delivered intervention for children with autism spectrum disorder living in regional Australia. J Autism Dev Disord. 2019;49:569–81.
54. Bearss K, Burrell TL, Challa SA, Postorino V, Gillespie SE, Crooks C, et al. Feasibility of parent training via telehealth for children with autism spectrum disorder and disruptive behavior: a demonstration pilot. J Autism Dev Disord. 2018;48(4):1020–30.

55. Aqdassi L, Sadeghi S, Pouretemad HR, Fathabadi JA. Family-based telerehabilitation program for improving gross motor skills in children with high functioning autism spectrum disorder. J Mod Rehabil. 2021;15(3):173–82.
56. Su WC, Cleffi C, Srinivasan S, Bhat A. Telehealth versus face-to-face fine motor and social communication interventions for children with autism spectrum disorder: efficacy, fidelity, acceptability, and feasibility. Am J Occup Ther. 2023;77(6):7706205130.
57. Lambert G, Alos N, Bernier P, et al. Patient and parent experiences with group telerehabilitation for child survivors of acute lymphoblastic leukemia. Int J Environ Res Public Health. 2021;18(7):3610.
58. Lambert G, Alos N, Bernier P, Laverdière C, Kairy D, Drummond K, et al. Home-based telehealth exercise intervention in early-on survivors of childhood acute lymphoblastic leukemia: feasibility study. JMIR Cancer. 2021;7(2):e25569.

9 Teleassessment Methods in Geriatric Rehabilitation

İsmet Tümtürk and Ferdi Başkurt

9.1 Introduction

Advancements in health science and technology are increasing life expectancy. The United Nations predicts that by 2050, one in six people will be over 65 years or older [1]. In addition, these advances are changing the way health services are administered to older adults [2]. Health services are increasingly delivered through remote methods [3]. Although the aging population is typically seen as a problem mainly affecting developed countries, the phenomenon of population aging is no longer limited to developed countries. There is an increasing percentage of older adults living in developed countries, and this rate will reach a global dimension in the coming years, including less developed countries [4]. Health problems inevitably increase with the cumulative decline in the physiological system with aging [5]. Additional health appointments after health problems increase the economic burden [6]. Furthermore, accessing health services is another barrier for older adults [7]. All these barriers are even more pronounced in extraordinary circumstances such as pandemics [8].

Therefore, the benefits of technology are even more important to keep the aging population more active. The use of self-assessment, telerehabilitation, and e-health methods in older adults improves the quality of life, facilitates access to health

İ. Tümtürk
Department of Physiotherapy and Rehabilitation, Institute of Health Sciences, Süleyman Demirel University, Isparta, Turkey

Department of Physiotherapy and Rehabilitation, Faculty of Health Sciences, Antalya Bilim University, Antalya, Turkey

F. Başkurt (✉)
Department of Physiotherapy and Rehabilitation, Faculty of Health Sciences, Süleyman Demirel University, Isparta, Turkey
e-mail: ferdibaskurt@sdu.edu.tr

F. Özden et al. (eds.), *Telerehabilitation*, TELe-Health,
https://doi.org/10.1007/978-3-031-69080-8_9

services, and minimizes various public health problems that may occur as a result of the aging of the population [9]. However, older adults may have barriers associated with telehealth use. Examples include technical literacy, ownership of technology, and mental acuity [10]. Therefore, the user and the caregiver must receive appropriate training on teleassessment and telehealth applications. Detailed knowledge of teleassessment methods by health professionals is necessary to explain these methods to users and caregivers [3]. This chapter presents teleassessment methods in geriatric rehabilitation.

9.2 Teleassessment in Geriatrics

9.2.1 Active and Healthy Aging and Teleassessment

Often, the main focus of technology research and development for older adults has been on the sick and disabled. However, focusing only on the sick older adult populations is a limited vision. The main issue is that older adults can age healthily and actively without disease with technology-based assessment [4]. World Health Organization defines "active aging" as "the process of developing and maintaining the functional ability that enables well-being in older age" [9]. Advances in communication technologies and teleassessment have great potential to improve the quality of life of older adults and enable active aging by assessing many parameters such as safety, mobility, independent living, vital signs, posture, and social participation [11]. Teleassessment methods are effective in terms of cost savings from health services, participation of the older adults in the community, keeping the older adults independent, aging properly, preventing possible aging-related falls, etc., and improving the quality of life of older adults [4]. There is now a need for a technological agenda that promotes active aging. The teleassessment methods presented in this chapter can provide timely and appropriate interventions to healthy older adults to maintain good health (Fig. 9.1).

Fig. 9.1 Teleassessment methods

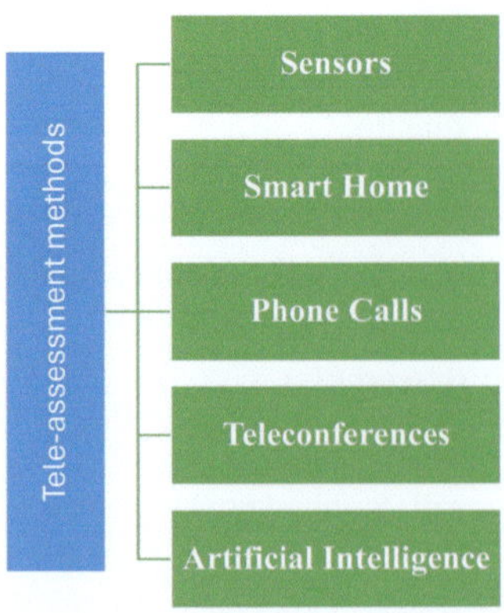

9.2.2 Sensors

How can health screenings with telehealth methods be done for chronically diseased or healthy older adults without inviting them to health institutions? Which teleassessment methods can assess older adults in their homes [12]? Data collected from sensors placed in the house, body-worn sensors, and sensors embedded in smartphones can be monitored to assess the health and well-being of older adults. These data can help identify new-onset health problems and provide feedback to older adults or their caregivers by detecting undesirable conditions such as abnormal posture and inactivity [4]. These sensors can monitor and transmit data on the body in real-time through their connection with tools such as the Internet of Things or mobile devices. Wearable sensors have rapidly evolved into advanced, multi-modal sensing devices that can assess parameters that monitor the wearer's mobility, vital signs, and even molecular data [13]. These physical sensors can monitor basic vital signs, heart rate, electrocardiogram, respiratory rate, body temperature, oxygen saturation, blood pressure, acceleration, postural sway, poor posture, muscle activity, gait parameters, anxiety level, limb movement directions, range of motion [3]. Wearable sensors monitor gait parameters, mobility, and other activity-related signals using motion sensors such as accelerometers or gyroscopes. Such wearables can detect fall incidents or assess gait disturbances in Parkinson's patients [3]. Fall risk assessment based on sensor technologies and data modeling methods has become a promising approach in older adults [14]. Hence, frequent hospital admissions are reduced [15]

Studies have noted improvements in the health of older adults through the transmission of blood pressure and body weight data to a remotely monitored server, and service providers have pointed out ease in monitoring health and preventing hospital readmissions [16, 17]. Blood pressure measurements can also be accurately measured with advanced smartwatches (Omron HeartGuide) [18]. Teleassessment and feedback systems in people with diabetes were also found to improve glycemic control, increase diabetes awareness, and improve quality of life. Patients monitored their blood glucose levels with sensors and transmitted their measurements via the Internet, and the provider evaluated the results and recommended dose titration via the Internet [19–22]. Bashshur et al. reported that the use of remote monitoring was superior to office visits across a wide range of conditions, including diabetes, hypertension, pain, cancer care, poststroke rehabilitation, and dementia [23].

Wearable sensors can also offer easy teleassessment. The accelerometer in a necklace allows monitoring of physical activity, including day and night. In addition, it can provide insights into resilience, depression, risk of falls, etc. [24]. Wearable sensors can also be employed to measure the joint motion angle of joints such as the knee, ankle, and trunk. It also measures parameters such as balance and gait. The locations of the sensors are thigh, lumbar, sternum, waist, insole, ankles, wrists, sacrum, L1 back level, T1 back level, abdomen, pelvis, head, calf, arms, and knee. The sensors used are an Inertial Measurement Unit, pressure, smart device, and electromyography (EMG) sensors [14, 25]. The relationship between a trunk range of motion based on a wearable inertial sensor and the fall risk of older people was assessed. The results showed that the non-falling group performed significantly better than the falling group on the average trunk range of motion across three body planes [26]. In other studies of Parkinson's patients, many parameters such as postural sway, parkour walking duration, number of steps, walking speed, step symmetry, cadence, arm oscillations, and trunk asymmetries could be measured with wearable sensors.

Moreover, the accuracy rates of these measurements were found at high levels [27]. These benefits of teleassessment methods are very crucial as it is known that the risk of falls and related problems is common in older adults [28]. Another aspect is the importance of sensors that receive location information and assessment technologies that can warn people with Alzheimer's disease if they leave the area where they live [29, 30].

Another type of sensor is a wearable chemical sensor. It is an essential milestone of such non-invasive chemical sensors that capture rich molecular data from the human body in real time. The use of wearable chemical sensors enables continuous, non-invasive monitoring of the dynamically changing chemical composition of various bioliquids such as sweat, tears, saliva, and interstitial fluid, thereby providing molecular-level insights into the health status of the wearer. These include monitoring dynamically changing glucose levels in diabetic patients, potassium ions in people with heart disease, and the stress hormone cortisol or the Parkinson's disease drug levodopa [31, 32]. The Oura Ring and VitalPatch systems are examples of recently introduced commercial, multi-parameter monitoring platforms that hold significant promise for remote geriatric care [33, 34]. With the development of smartwatch technology, these measurements are becoming simpler.

Non-wearable sensor types are also available. There is also a growing interest in non-wearable sensors based on smart home digital systems to monitor data such as the posture, range of motion, and activity of older adults. These sensors can analyze data and alert caregivers or health professionals of any abnormalities, thus supporting the health and safety of older adults in their homes. For example, some studies use the Kinect camera as a sensor to assess the mobility and gait of older adults in their homes [35, 36].

9.2.3 Smart Home

Smart home applications for older adults enable the emergence of smart homes with extended surveillance and communication systems that can be assessed at any time, helping them to live healthy and independent lives. Such smart homes for older adults can convert various body-worn sensors and electronic surveillance devices into home monitoring systems via a wireless communication network. These systems continuously monitor the health and activities of older adults and remotely inform caregivers or healthcare professionals about abnormal changes. Smart home designs should be adapted depending on the frailty of older adults and chronic conditions such as diabetes, heart disease, or kidney disease. Different types of sensors, distributed throughout the home or worn on the body, can detect movement in specific locations. Smart socks, insoles, shoes, mirrors, or carpets can evaluate gait, balance, foot problems, and fragility. For example, the data collected from motion sensors distributed in digital mirrors can assess body posture, joint range of motion, or even a fall event [37]. They can also be audio-visual displays (e.g., appointments or medication reminders). Systems such as Amazon Echo or Google Home also help detect emergencies through continuous monitoring and provide personalized medication reminders and social and cognitive stimulation. Other parts of the smart home, such as the kitchen or bathroom, contribute to the surveillance of older adults' health, daily activities, and nutrition, using digital systems such as smart refrigerators (which keep track of stored food or medicines) or smart toilets (which analyze urine or feces) [3].

In summary, smart homes can consist of: (a) standalone objects that operate intelligently (e.g., smart locks), (b) connected smart objects that share information (e.g., sensors, smart home hubs, controllers), (c) remote interactive and automated systems that may include data collection, (d) technologies that use collected data to adapt to the future needs of older adults (e.g., machine learning), (e) technologies that can continuously collect data [38]. According to a review study, five types of smart home technology systems have been utilized: Dem@Care project, Rosetta system, Technology Integrated Health Management system, Night Monitoring System, and Home-Based Technologies with Teleassistance System. Dem@Care is a sensor-based system for cognitive and functional status. The Rosetta System is a fully integrated multifunctional modular system combining assistive technologies. Technology Integrated Health Management System is a continuous remote monitoring system through sensors, vital signs monitors, and GPS tracking devices. Night Monitoring System includes a control panel, wireless receiver, motion, door and bed sensors, text, voice, and alarm sounds. Home-based technologies with Teleassistance Systems include a night light pathway, remote intercom, electronic bracelet, and central telephone hotline [38].

Smart homes use environmental sensors such as infrared motion, contact, light, temperature, and humidity to enable monitoring of older adults' movements. Infrared sensors can provide information on older adults' location, time spent in a single room, frequency of toilet use, and sleep status. These detectors are often used to monitor the Activity of Daily Living. Contact sensors can provide information that a door is open or closed. Door usage patterns provide information about older adults entering and leaving the home. Light sensors placed throughout the home provide information on the ambient light level in each room throughout the day, providing indirect data on older adults' activity levels during the day or night. For example, light sensors inside the refrigerator provide information on food-related routines. The combination of sensors that detect temperature, humidity, and motion can give information on daily activities [39]. Smart homes additionally provide different types of data such as electrocardiogram, pulse, blood pressure, etc., detection of events in the home, fall detection, and interactions with virtual assistants. Smart home environments have great potential to support older adults. Robot-assisted smart homes and assessments will also be a focus in the future [40].

The results of studies using smart homes on older adults have provided some evidence of positive impact (in terms of improved physical activity, activities of daily living, sleep, anxiety, depression, agitation, irritability, cognitive functioning, falls, nocturnal injuries, and unattended home exits) [38]. Studies report that smart homes help participants stay active [41, 42]. A recent review reported that smart home technologies show great potential in managing chronic diseases at home. Smart homes also improve the quality of life of older adults. Furthermore, the review emphasizes that smart homes enable continuous monitoring of older adults by health professionals [39]. However, in most studies, privacy, lack of human contact, loss of usefulness and autonomy, and intrusiveness are obstacles for smart home users [43]. Privacy was not a concern for older adults as long as the data collected in a study exploring users' experiences was only available to family members, caregivers, or health professionals [44].

9.2.4 Phone Calls and Teleconferences

The first step in telerehabilitation is remote assessment. With a proper patient assessment, it is possible to establish a functional baseline for the patient, evaluate the effectiveness of treatment, and integrate data to measure progress. The core component of every assessment is the patient interview, which can be completed through remote evaluations. In addition, with some creative adaptations and the application of technology, a comprehensive physical examination can be performed, including observation, movement examinations, standardized tests, specific tests, and range of motion. Telehealth can also be applied to assess older adults in remote areas by sending and receiving information via phone calls, text messaging services, media messaging services, the Internet, etc. For example, the addition of videoconferencing provides a more cost-effective outcome for assessment and maintenance [9]. The studies demonstrated good validity in terms of the feasibility of measuring pain, swelling, range of motion, muscle strength, balance, gait, and functional outcomes. Inter-rater and intra-rater reliability showed excellent levels of telerehabilitation for low back pain, ankle disorders, elbow disorders, total knee replacement, and non-articular lower limb disorders [45, 46]. The presence of a family member or caregiver during teleconferencing sessions is also essential for people with severe disabilities. Informed consent should be obtained in advance. Patients should be trained to choose a comfortable and quiet place for their visit. The combination of audio/visual conferencing with wearable sensors has been evaluated and shown to improve the quality of measurements [47, 48]. During teleconferencing sessions, it may be helpful for participants to use home appliances to take measurements such as temperature, heart rate, blood pressure, weight, and blood sugar [9].

Specialized assessment questionnaires can also be administered to older adults, such as patient-reported outcome measures via teleconferencing and mobile application techniques [49–51]. In addition, activities of daily living, cognitive assessment, assessment of depression and psychological states, nutritional assessment, fall frequency and risk assessment, caregiver burden assessment, and social and environmental issues can be assessed by teleconferencing [52]. Inspectional evaluations such as posture and range of motion can also be performed in older adults thanks to video interviews with developing camera systems [52–54]. A recent meta-analysis explored the effects of video teleconsultations in primary care and mental health services. The findings suggest that videoconferencing offers a convenient and effective alternative [55].

Observation of a patient's gait is relatively simple with videoconferencing technology. Palpation, on the other hand, cannot be done by teleassessment; instead, the patient can be asked to participate in self-palpation with real-time demonstration and verbal guidance from the clinician [56]. Movement examinations are another challenge due to the lack of clinic-based measurement tools; however, specialized rehabilitation tools have been designed, such as the "eHAB" videoconferencing technology that integrates videoconferencing, measurement, media tools, and assessment protocols [57]. Specific testing of muscles, nerves, or joints can pose another challenge, but at-home caregivers and family members can perform the tests with guidance from the clinician. Other tests, such as range of motion, can be done in real time, allowing accurate anthropometric measurements using optics to detect joints. Motion sensors and body monitoring technology have evolved [58, 59]. Also, OPTI-RERC is a project that provides home-based motor assessment, optimizing participation through technology for successful aging. There are also commercially available technologies such as the "Sony Eyetoy". This system analyzes upper and lower limb movements and balance [60]. Other examples include "AMMR" mixed reality rehabilitation and "Mercury", a wearable sensor network platform for high-accuracy motion analysis [61].

9.2.5 Artificial Intelligence

Meeting the challenge of large amounts of dynamic data, continuously collected from multiple sources, requires a multi-disciplinary approach to big data processing and analysis. Therefore, it is essential to use machine learning or artificial intelligence techniques for decision-making, speeding up diagnoses, and combining and interpreting data [3]. The smart vest and an advanced wearable with embedded sensors enable the collection of a lot of data from the wearer. The potential for using the Internet of Things, machine learning, and artificial intelligence is growing [62]. These technologies are used to assess and treat many medical conditions [62]. The studies show remarkable promise for diagnosing patients with neurocognitive disorders through artificial intelligence technology [63]. According to a review, the most common artificial intelligence devices used were robots, exoskeleton devices, smart homes, artificial intelligence-powered smart health apps and wearables, voice-activated devices, and virtual reality [64]. In the studies, participants' location, activity intensity, sleep patterns, mood, social interaction, medication use, physiological indicators and vital signs were monitored with the support of artificial intelligence [64, 65]. As a result, these systems show potential for supporting independent living, reducing falls among older adults, detecting various long-term conditions early, and more [66].

9.3 Teleassessment Difficulties in Older Adults

Older adults with digital literacy difficulties and visual impairments may need help using mobile devices or teleassessment methods with many buttons, small text, and poor color contrast. Therefore, it would be more beneficial to extend digital health services to the geriatric population and develop more accessible, user-specific methods with fewer buttons, larger text, and improved color contrast. Devices need to be user-centered so that people with hearing impairments or other health conditions can continue to use and benefit from them. It is also essential that systems such as AI smart homes are more accessible and less costly. The longevity of devices, device size, and weight are also crucial for the technological revolution in health [3]. Improved network coverage at affordable prices is also critical for impactful telemedicine activities, especially in rural areas [3]. In addition, as mentioned above, ethical considerations are also important. However, these issues are covered elsewhere in the present book.

9.4 Conclusion

Almost all outcome measures measured during a traditional office-based physical examination can now be measured remotely during virtual visits [3]. Teleassessment can be used in the follow-up of older adults with many conditions, such as chronic pain, spinal stenosis, stroke, amputation, Parkinson's disease, and dementia. Older adults need to be assessed for fall risk. With teleassessment (e.g., mobile apps, teleconferences, sensors), fall risk can be assessed frequently and effortlessly. For example, in one study, the Berg Balance Scale was applied with teleassessment methods, which was reported to be reliable and possible. However, it was emphasized that multidimensional advanced camera systems and slow-motion technology should be used for such evaluations [43, 62]. The feasibility of measuring pain, swelling, range of motion, muscle strength, balance, gait, and functional outcomes was demonstrated with good concurrent validity. Inter-rater and intra-rater reliability was excellent for teleassessment in various diseases [46].

A combined approach should be used, following recent new developments in teleassessment methods. During assessments, a multi-personal approach should be realized with the support of caregivers and other health professionals. Teleassessment sessions should be designed according to ethical guidelines and difficulties of use. This chapter presents teleassessment methods offered by emerging technology and provides information for health professionals.

References

1. Cai Y, Song W, Li J, Jing Y, Liang C, Zhang L, et al. The landscape of aging. Sci China Life Sci. 2022;65(12):2354–454. https://doi.org/10.1007/s11427-022-2161-3.

2. Oh-Park M, Lew HL, Raghavan P. Telerehabilitation for geriatrics. Phys Med Rehabil Clin. 2021;32(2):291–305. https://doi.org/10.1016/j.pmr.2021.01.003.
3. Chen C, Ding S, Wang J. Digital health for aging populations. Nat Med. 2023;29(7):1623–30. https://doi.org/10.1038/s41591-023-02391-8.
4. Sixsmith A. Technology and the challenge of aging. In: Sixsmith A, Gutman G, editors. Technologies for active aging. Boston: Springer; 2013. p. 7–25.
5. Wang X, Hu J, Wu D. Risk factors for frailty in older adults. Medicine (Baltimore). 2022;101(34):e30169. https://doi.org/10.1097/md.0000000000030169.
6. Picco L, Achilla E, Abdin E, Chong SA, Vaingankar JA, McCrone P, et al. Economic burden of multimorbidity among older adults: impact on healthcare and societal costs. BMC Health Serv Res. 2016;16(1):173. https://doi.org/10.1186/s12913-016-1421-7.
7. Wolfe MK, McDonald NC, Holmes GM. Transportation barriers to health care in the United States: findings from the National Health Interview Survey, 1997–2017. Am J Public Health. 2020;110(6):815–22. https://doi.org/10.2105/AJPH.2020.305579.
8. Oluyede L, Cochran AL, Wolfe M, Prunkl L, McDonald N. Addressing transportation barriers to health care during the COVID-19 pandemic: perspectives of care coordinators. Transp Res A Policy Pract. 2022;159:157–68. https://doi.org/10.1016/j.tra.2022.03.010.
9. Dionyssiotis Y. Telerehabilitation in geriatrics. In: Alexander M, editor. Telerehabilitation. New Delhi: Elsevier; 2022. p. 149–60.
10. Kruse C, Fohn J, Wilson N, Nunez Patlan E, Zipp S, Mileski M. Utilization barriers and medical outcomes commensurate with the use of telehealth among older adults: systematic review. JMIR Med Inform. 2020;8(8):e20359. https://doi.org/10.2196/20359.
11. Sixsmith A, Gutman G. Introduction. In: Sixsmith A, Gutman G, editors. Technologies for active aging. Boston: Springer; 2013. p. 1–5.
12. Wiles JL, Leibing A, Guberman N, Reeve J, Allen RES. The meaning of "aging in place" to older people. The Gerontologist. 2012;52(3):357–66. https://doi.org/10.1093/geront/gnr098.
13. Sim I. Mobile devices and health. N Engl J Med. 2019;381(10):956–68. https://doi.org/10.1056/NEJMra1806949.
14. Chen M, Wang H, Yu L, Yeung EH, Luo J, Tsui K-L, et al. A systematic review of wearable sensor-based technologies for fall risk assessment in older adults. Sensors. 2022;22(18):6752. https://doi.org/10.3390/s22186752.
15. Foster MV, Sethares KA. Facilitators and barriers to the adoption of telehealth in older adults: an integrative review. Comput Inform Nurs. 2014;32(11):523–33.
16. Dar O, Riley J, Chapman C, Dubrey SW, Morris S, Rosen SD, et al. A randomized trial of home telemonitoring in a typical elderly heart failure population in North West London: results of the Home-HF study. Eur J Heart Fail. 2009;11(3):319–25. https://doi.org/10.1093/eurjhf/hfn050.
17. Czaja SJ, Lee CC, Arana N, Nair SN, Sharit J. Use of a telehealth system by older adults with hypertension. J Telemed Telecare. 2014;20(4):184–91. https://doi.org/10.1177/1357633X14533889.
18. Vaseekaran M, Kaese S, Görlich D, Wiemer M, Samol A. WATCH–BPM–comparison of a WATCH-type blood pressure monitor with a conventional ambulatory blood pressure monitor and auscultatory sphygmomanometry. Sensors. 2023;23(21):8877. https://doi.org/10.3390/s23218877.
19. Jaana M, Paré G. Home telemonitoring of patients with diabetes: a systematic assessment of observed effects. J Eval Clin Pract. 2007;13(2):242–53. https://doi.org/10.1111/j.1365-2753.2006.00686.x.
20. Verhoeven F, van Gemert-Pijnen L, Dijkstra K, Nijland N, Seydel E, Steehouder M. The contribution of teleconsultation and videoconferencing to diabetes care: a systematic literature review. J Med Internet Res. 2007;9(5):e37. https://doi.org/10.2196/jmir.9.5.e37.
21. Bujnowska-Fedak MM, Puchała E, Steciwko A. The impact of telehome care on health status and quality of life among patients with diabetes in a primary care setting in Poland. Telemed eHealth. 2011;17(3):153–63. https://doi.org/10.1089/tmj.2010.0113.
22. Prato SD, Nicolucci A, Lovagnini-Scher AC, Turco S, Leotta S, Vespasiani G, et al. Telecare provides comparable efficacy to conventional self-monitored blood glucose in patients with

type 2 diabetes titrating one injection of insulin glulisine—the ELEONOR study. Diabetes Technol Ther. 2011;14(2):175–82. https://doi.org/10.1089/dia.2011.0163.
23. Bashshur RL, Shannon GW, Smith BR, Alverson DC, Antoniotti N, Barsan WG, et al. The empirical foundations of telemedicine interventions for chronic disease management. Telemed eHealth. 2014;20(9):769–800. https://doi.org/10.1089/tmj.2014.9981.
24. Razjouyan J, Naik AD, Horstman MJ, Kunik ME, Amirmazaheri M, Zhou H, et al. Wearable sensors and the assessment of frailty among vulnerable older adults: an observational cohort study. Sensors. 2018;18(5):1336. https://doi.org/10.3390/s18051336.
25. Díaz S, Stephenson JB, Labrador MA. Use of wearable sensor technology in gait, balance, and range of motion analysis. Appl Sci. 2020;10(1):234. https://doi.org/10.3390/app10010234.
26. Yu X, Park S, Xiong S. Trunk range of motion: a wearable sensor-based test protocol and indicator of fall risk in older people. Appl Ergon. 2023;108:103963. https://doi.org/10.1016/j.apergo.2023.103963.
27. Balakrishnan A, Medikonda J, Namboothiri PK, Manik M, Natarajan A. Role of wearable sensors with machine learning approaches in gait analysis for Parkinson's disease assessment: a review. Eng Sci. 2022;19:5–19. https://doi.org/10.30919/es8e622.
28. Hsieh Katherine L, Chen L, Sosnoff Jacob J. Mobile technology for falls prevention in older adults. J Gerontol. 2023;78(5):861–8. https://doi.org/10.1093/gerona/glac116.
29. García-Requejo A, Pérez-Rubio MC, Villadangos JM, Hernández Á. Activity monitoring and location sensory system for people with mild cognitive impairments. IEEE Sensors J. 2023;23(5):5448–58. https://doi.org/10.1109/JSEN.2023.3239980.
30. Pai M-C, Jan S-S. Have I been here? Sense of location in people with Alzheimer's disease. Front Aging Neurosci. 2020;12:582525. https://doi.org/10.3389/fnagi.2020.582525.
31. Kim J, Campbell AS, de Ávila BE-F, Wang J. Wearable biosensors for healthcare monitoring. Nat Biotechnol. 2019;37(4):389–406. https://doi.org/10.1038/s41587-019-0045-y.
32. Sempionatto JR, Lasalde-Ramírez JA, Mahato K, Wang J, Gao W. Wearable chemical sensors for biomarker discovery in the omics era. Nat Rev Chem. 2022;6(12):899–915. https://doi.org/10.1038/s41570-022-00439-w.
33. Grifantini K. Tracking sleep to optimize health. IEEE Pulse. 2020;11(5):12–6. https://doi.org/10.1109/MPULS.2020.3022142.
34. Tonino RPB, Larimer K, Eissen O, Schipperus MR. Remote patient monitoring in adults receiving transfusion or infusion for hematological disorders using the VitalPatch and accelerateIQ monitoring system: quantitative feasibility study. JMIR Hum Factors. 2019;6(4):e15103. https://doi.org/10.2196/15103.
35. Momin MS, Sufian A, Barman D, Dutta P, Dong M, Leo M. In-home older adults' activity pattern monitoring using depth sensors: a review. Sensors. 2022;22(23):9067. https://doi.org/10.3390/s22239067.
36. Liu Y, Zhang G, Tarolli CG, Hristov R, Jensen-Roberts S, Waddell EM, et al. Monitoring gait at home with radio waves in Parkinson's disease: a marker of severity, progression, and medication response. Sci Transl Med. 2022;14(663):eadc9669.
37. Miotto R, Danieletto M, Scelza JR, Kidd BA, Dudley JT. Reflecting health: smart mirrors for personalized medicine. NPJ Digit Med. 2018;1(1):62. https://doi.org/10.1038/s41746-018-0068-7.
38. Moyle W, Murfield J, Lion K. The effectiveness of smart home technologies to support the health outcomes of community-dwelling older adults living with dementia: a scoping review. Int J Med Inform. 2021;153:104513. https://doi.org/10.1016/j.ijmedinf.2021.104513.
39. Facchinetti G, Petrucci G, Albanesi B, De Marinis MG, Piredda M. Can smart home technologies help older adults manage their chronic condition? A systematic literature review. Int J Environ Res Public Health. 2023;20(2):1205. https://doi.org/10.3390/ijerph20021205.
40. Ghafurian M, Wang K, Dhode I, Kapoor M, Morita PP, Dautenhahn K. Smart home devices for supporting older adults: a systematic review. IEEE Access. 2023;11:47137–58. https://doi.org/10.1109/ACCESS.2023.3266647.
41. Lie ML, Lindsay S, Brittain K. Technology and trust: older people's perspectives of a home monitoring system. Ageing Soc. 2016;36(7):1501–25.

42. Pol M, van Nes F, van Hartingsveldt M, Buurman B, de Rooij S, Kröse B. Older people's perspectives regarding the use of sensor monitoring in their home. The Gerontologist. 2016;56(3):485–93. https://doi.org/10.1093/geront/gnu104.
43. Ghorayeb A, Comber R, Gooberman-Hill R. Older adults' perspectives of smart home technology: are we developing the technology that older people want? Int J Hum Comput Stud. 2021;147:102571. https://doi.org/10.1016/j.ijhcs.2020.102571.
44. Bock C, Demiris G, Choi Y, Le T, Thompson HJ, Samuel A, et al. Engaging older adults in the visualization of sensor data facilitated by an open platform for connected devices. Technol Health Care. 2016;24:541–50. https://doi.org/10.3233/THC-161150.
45. Lee AC, Davenport TE, Randall K. Telehealth physical therapy in musculoskeletal practice. J Orthop Sports Phys Ther. 2018;48(10):736–9. https://doi.org/10.2519/jospt.2018.0613.
46. Mani S, Sharma S, Omar B, Paungmali A, Joseph L. Validity and reliability of Internet-based physiotherapy assessment for musculoskeletal disorders: a systematic review. J Telemed Telecare. 2016;23(3):379–91. https://doi.org/10.1177/1357633X16642369.
47. Winters JM, Wang Y, Winters JM. Wearable sensors and telerehabilitation. IEEE Eng Med Biol Mag. 2003;22(3):56–65.
48. Zheng H, Black ND, Harris ND. Position-sensing technologies for movement analysis in stroke rehabilitation. Med Biol Eng Comput. 2005;43(4):413–20. https://doi.org/10.1007/BF02344720.
49. Narasimha S, Madathil KC, Agnisarman S, Rogers H, Welch B, Ashok A, et al. Designing telemedicine systems for geriatric patients: a review of the usability studies. Telemed eHealth. 2016;23(6):459–72. https://doi.org/10.1089/tmj.2016.0178.
50. DiGiovanni G, Mousaw K, Lloyd T, Dukelow N, Fitzgerald B, D'Aurizio H, et al. Development of a telehealth geriatric assessment model in response to the COVID-19 pandemic. J Geriatr Oncol. 2020;11(5):761–3. https://doi.org/10.1016/j.jgo.2020.04.007.
51. Thompson LI, Harrington KD, Roque N, Strenger J, Correia S, Jones RN, et al. A highly feasible, reliable, and fully remote protocol for mobile app-based cognitive assessment in cognitively healthy older adults. Alzheimers Dement. 2022;14(1):e12283. https://doi.org/10.1002/dad2.12283.
52. Sabo A, Mehdizadeh S, Ng K-D, Iaboni A, Taati B. Assessment of Parkinsonian gait in older adults with dementia via human pose tracking in video data. J Neuroeng Rehabil. 2020;17(1):97. https://doi.org/10.1186/s12984-020-00728-9.
53. Steinert A, Sattler I, Otte K, Röhling H, Mansow-Model S, Müller-Werdan U. Using new camera-based technologies for gait analysis in older adults in comparison to the established GAITRite system. Sensors. 2019;20(1):125. https://doi.org/10.3390/s20010125.
54. Dawe RJ, Yu L, Leurgans SE, Truty T, Curran T, Hausdorff JM, et al. Expanding instrumented gait testing in the community setting: a portable, depth-sensing camera captures joint motion in older adults. PLoS One. 2019;14(5):e0215995. https://doi.org/10.1371/journal.pone.0215995.
55. Carrillo de Albornoz S, Sia K-L, Harris A. The effectiveness of teleconsultations in primary care: systematic review. Fam Pract. 2022;39(1):168–82. https://doi.org/10.1093/fampra/cmab077.
56. Fiani B, Siddiqi I, Lee SC, Dhillon L. Telerehabilitation: development, application, and need for increased usage in the COVID-19 era for patients with spinal pathology. Cureus. 2020;12(9):e10563. https://doi.org/10.7759/cureus.10563.
57. Peel NM, Russell TG, Gray LC. Feasibility of using an in-home video conferencing system in geriatric rehabilitation. J Rehabil Med. 2011;43(4):364–6. https://doi.org/10.2340/16501977-0675.
58. Dent PA, Wilke B, Terkonda S, Luther I, Shi GG. Validation of teleconference-based goniometry for measuring elbow joint range of motion. Cureus. 2020;12(2):e6925. https://doi.org/10.7759/cureus.6925.
59. Porciuncula F, Roto AV, Kumar D, Davis I, Roy S, Walsh CJ, et al. Wearable movement sensors for rehabilitation: a focused review of technological and clinical advances. PM R. 2018;10(9S2):S220–32. https://doi.org/10.1016/j.pmrj.2018.06.013.

60. Lange BS, Requejo P, Flynn SM, Rizzo AA, Valero-Cuevas FJ, Baker L, et al. The potential of virtual reality and gaming to assist successful aging with disability. Phys Med Rehabil Clin. 2010;21(2):339–56. https://doi.org/10.1016/j.pmr.2009.12.007.
61. Altilio R, Liparulo L, Panella M, Proietti A, Paoloni M. Multimedia and gaming technologies for telerehabilitation of motor disabilities [leading edge]. IEEE Technol Soc Mag. 2015;34(4):23–30. https://doi.org/10.1109/MTS.2015.2494279.
62. Venkataraman K, Morgan M, Amis KA, Landerman LR, Koh GC, Caves K, et al. Teleassessment of the berg balance scale: effects of transmission characteristics. Arch Phys Med Rehabil. 2017;98(4):659–64.e1. https://doi.org/10.1016/j.apmr.2016.10.019.
63. Graham SA, Lee EE, Jeste DV, Van Patten R, Twamley EW, Nebeker C, et al. Artificial intelligence approaches to predicting and detecting cognitive decline in older adults: a conceptual review. Psychiatry Res. 2020;284:112732. https://doi.org/10.1016/j.psychres.2019.112732.
64. Ma B, Yang J, Wong FKY, Wong AKC, Ma T, Meng J, et al. Artificial intelligence in elderly healthcare: a scoping review. Ageing Res Rev. 2023;83:101808. https://doi.org/10.1016/j.arr.2022.101808.
65. Lee C-H, Wang C, Fan X, Li F, Chen C-H. Artificial intelligence-enabled digital transformation in elderly healthcare field: scoping review. Adv Eng Inform. 2023;55:101874. https://doi.org/10.1016/j.aei.2023.101874.
66. Baig MM, Afifi S, GholamHosseini H, Mirza F. A systematic review of wearable sensors and IoT-based monitoring applications for older adults—a focus on ageing population and independent living. J Med Syst. 2019;43(8):233. https://doi.org/10.1007/s10916-019-1365-7.

10 Telerehabilitation Methods in Geriatric Rehabilitation

Onur Aydoğdu

10.1 Geriatrics: Aging of the Population

A person 65 years and older is generally considered a geriatric individual [1]. The geriatric population in the world is steadily increasing day by day [2]. In addition, the world population is getting older every day. In 2050, it is estimated that the proportion of people over 60 will reach 22% of the entire population, and one in four people living in Europe and North America will be geriatric [3]. Similarly, Southeast Asian countries are also facing the problem of aging. The number of geriatric individuals in this region is expected to increase from approximately 250 million in 2019 to 570 million in 2050 [4]. The increase in the geriatric population is expected to be worldwide; for example, in Greece, it is expected to be around 50% [3].

This rapid increase in the aging of society has occurred, especially in recent years. The worldwide geriatric population is estimated to increase by 65% in 2030 compared to 2015 and reach 1.4 billion people from 900 million. It is thought that this increase will also affect the population aged 80 years and over, and the number of people aged 80 years and over worldwide is expected to increase from 120 million in 2015 to approximately 450 million in 2050 [3]. Worldwide, geriatric individuals aged 85 years and over are projected to increase by more than 350% between 2010 and 2050 [5].

When we look at the worldwide population values, the USA has the largest geriatric population among developed countries. According to the 2012 census, the number of geriatric individuals in the USA was approximately 45 million, expected to reach approximately 85 million in 2050. The geriatric population in the USA is

O. Aydoğdu (✉)
Department of Physiotherapy and Rehabilitation, Faculty of Health Sciences, Marmara University, Istanbul, Turkey
e-mail: onur.aydogdu@marmara.edu.tr

F. Özden et al. (eds.), *Telerehabilitation*, TELe-Health,
https://doi.org/10.1007/978-3-031-69080-8_10

increasing steadily and is estimated to be one in five of the entire population in 2030 [6].

The worrying situation for the geriatric population is that the levels of chronic diseases and dependency increase as individuals age [7]. With aging, some biopsychosocial changes occur in the individual; frailty is encountered, and the incidence of degenerative diseases and functional dependence increases [2]. With the aging of society, the level of comorbidity and frailty increases, the level of physical activity decreases, and functional impairments such as disability and poor quality of life occur [4].

Chronic and systemic diseases leading to functional disabilities decrease the quality of life of geriatric individuals and increase the cost of care [7]. Geriatric individuals prone to frailty bring additional burdens and costs to healthcare systems [4]. A significant portion (approximately 70%) of health expenditures in the USA is for the geriatric population. In 2005, 1.3 trillion dollars were spent on the geriatric population, estimated to have doubled (2.5 trillion dollars) in 2014 [7]. In the United States, most of the resources allocated for health services are spent on treating chronic and systemic diseases such as heart diseases, diabetes, and rheumatological diseases that geriatric individuals have [8]. Sustainable, manageable strategies are required to combat this worldwide health problem [4]. The issue of reducing hospitalizations with aging has encouraged health legislators to use rehabilitation resources more effectively and appropriately [9].

The growing geriatric population and its increasing proportion in society attract the attention of politicians and legislators, and initiatives are being taken to address this [6]. The number of elderly people worldwide has made the need for rehabilitation in geriatric individuals the focus of health policy and clinical research [9]. As the population ages, the need for specialized facilities and home care for geriatric individuals will increase [5]. As the number of patients worldwide increases, there is a need for effective and better rehabilitation services [10]. Due to the increasing aging population and the increasing need for physiotherapy and rehabilitation practices, health professionals must provide safe, evidence-based, beneficial options [11].

10.2 Rehabilitation in Geriatrics

Some of the most basic problems of geriatric individuals are their chronic diseases and their need for care [6]. Chronic diseases are the main problems that lead to a decrease in the activities of daily living and quality of life of geriatric individuals [12]. Decreased physical capacity negatively affects the functional capacity of frail geriatric individuals [13]. In 2016, just over 50% of geriatric individuals in Greece reported that they were physically limited due to a health problem [3]. On the other hand, these negative effects can be prevented with regular training sessions, and falls, common in geriatric individuals, can be prevented [13]. Therefore, health professionals should be involved alongside the elderly for a qualified aging process [2].

The definition of being healthy in elderly individuals is not only the absence of the effects of diseases but also the preservation of functional independence in their daily lives [2]. Regular therapeutic exercises, one of the key points for a healthy aging process, are an important component of physiotherapy and rehabilitation practices [11]. As a branch of therapeutic exercises, regular physical activity plays an important role in geriatric individuals in terms of staying healthy and reducing the effects of changes brought by aging. Regular physical activity contributes to the neuromuscular system in addition to the cardiovascular system [2].

Hip fractures are one of the most common conditions in geriatric individuals that require rehabilitation. Hip fractures are one of the most serious problems seen in geriatric individuals, leading to negative psychological effects in addition to functional limitation and disability. Hip fractures, which reduce the level of functional independence and quality of life and restrict activities of daily living, are among the most common injuries in geriatric individuals. As the number of geriatric individuals increases, hip fractures also increase. It is estimated that 2.5 million geriatric individuals will have hip fracture problems every year in 2025, and more than six million geriatric individuals will have hip fracture problems every year in 2050 [3]. In addition to hip fractures, another common problem in geriatric individuals is total hip arthroplasty. It is reported that geriatric patients stay in the hospital for an average of 2 weeks after total hip arthroplasty. Still, the most important part of rehabilitation is performed outside the hospital. Some clinicians suggest that the optimal duration of rehabilitation after total hip arthroplasty may start from the first postoperative day and last up to 6 months [14]. After hospitalization, the gait functions of approximately two-thirds of geriatric patients may deteriorate. While half of geriatric individuals are dependent on walking, approximately one-fifth are not mobile [15]. As a consequence, geriatric individuals with such chronic and systemic conditions and disabled people request to receive their treatment sessions by staying at home [8]. Rapid discharge, home care, and geriatric rehabilitation are recommended for such individuals [9].

Comorbidities and acute diseases are among the most important factors that lead to demand for geriatric rehabilitation programs [12]. Due to all these problems, geriatric individuals need comprehensive rehabilitation [15]. A good rehabilitation should be progressive, individualized, and have a comprehensive protocol [14]. Consequently, it is known that more people worldwide need health services, especially physiotherapy and rehabilitation, every year [3].

Geriatric rehabilitation is defined as multidimensional diagnostic and therapeutic interventions to maintain functional capacity, increase social participation, and promote activity in elderly individuals with disabilities. Geriatric rehabilitation consists of a multidisciplinary care and health service [9]. Geriatric rehabilitation is an important component of health services that geriatric individuals need for many diseases and conditions that may be experienced due to aging. Increasing functional capacity, restoring physical activity, and encouraging socialization are among the main objectives of geriatric rehabilitation. Geriatric rehabilitation combines multidimensional practices for diagnosis and treatment [16].

Although they do not receive specialized treatment, many geriatric individuals require comprehensive therapeutic interventions. The limited treatment options available to some geriatric individuals are inpatient, outpatient, and home health care [7]. The main aim of geriatric rehabilitation in a hospital or clinical center is for the older person to return home. However, the return home of geriatric patients does not necessarily mean they are fully recovered [9]. Health expenditures can be reduced by discharging patients earlier and providing care services at home [7]. Rehabilitation sessions in the postoperative period are usually followed as outpatient/at home due to rapid postoperative recovery, short hospital stays, and the COVID-19 outbreak [17]. In China, rehabilitation is mainly performed by telephone or outpatient visits. However, some rehabilitation practices cannot be applied correctly by telephone [14]. In discharged geriatric patients, limitations in activities of daily living and functional dependence persist in some cases, so home rehabilitation is of considerable importance for geriatric individuals. Geriatric individuals have reported high satisfaction with home rehabilitation [9]. Home-based telerehabilitation is monitoring patients in their homes from a health center such as a hospital or clinic [7]. Home-based rehabilitation is a rehabilitation method that aims to follow rehabilitation practices from home instead of the hospital. Common types of home-based rehabilitation are telephone follow-ups and regular hospital outpatient reviews [17]. The main aim of home-based telerehabilitation is to improve healthcare services, reduce care costs, and monitor the patient from home [7]. On the other hand, the disadvantages of home-based rehabilitation services are the inability to follow the patient regularly, lack of easy access to information about his/her medical condition, transportation difficulties, and transportation costs [6]. The adherence of geriatric patients to home exercise programs is also generally low [10]. It has been reported that health professionals in rural areas have insufficient professional knowledge and an imbalance in access to rehabilitation practices [12]. It has also been documented that many geriatric patients living in geographically isolated areas or areas with limited health services face limitations in accessing the rehabilitation interventions they need at the right time [10].

The COVID-19 outbreak has greatly affected healthcare services due to restrictions to ensure the safety of healthcare professionals and patients [18]. COVID-19 disease, which disrupts healthcare services worldwide, causes greater problems for geriatric individuals. Geriatric individuals are the most susceptible population affected by COVID-19 disease. While many geriatric individuals could not access rehabilitation services for some reasons before the COVID-19 pandemic, this number increased even more during the pandemic and isolation periods [12]. The coronavirus pandemic, which started in 2019, led healthcare professionals and patients to a different healthcare option [6].

There is an increase in demand for healthcare services among geriatric individuals. Therefore, health professionals and providers know this demand and propose up-to-date, innovative practices [10]. Recent information technology advances have significantly changed how healthcare services are provided [19]. Due to the aging of the population worldwide and the advancement of technology, innovations are occurring in the delivery of healthcare services. In this context, telerehabilitation is a promising potential modality [20]. More and more countries are demanding their citizens switch to digital systems. Although this is difficult for them, it is also valid for geriatric individuals [13]. In light of all this information, there is a need for methods where rehabilitation practices are carried out through telephone calls or videoconferencing without the need for face-to-face meetings in hospitals or clinical centers [10].

In conclusion, health professionals, politicians, and legislators are seeking and developing more efficient and cost-effective systems that promote independence and provide treatment for the elderly at home [8]. With the increase in the elderly population in society, the convergence of health and technology, and the increasing number of people in need of rehabilitation, various innovations have been provided to increase efficiency and reduce costs in health services [16]. Telerehabilitation, a method used to maintain therapeutic exercises [2], may be an important modality for healthcare professionals. As a result, telerehabilitation may be an alternative method to offer face-to-face exercise to geriatric individuals who cannot receive physiotherapy and rehabilitation services due to the problems mentioned above [11]. For all these reasons, telerehabilitation has become more important and popular for geriatric individuals [12].

10.3 Technology in Geriatrics (Gerontechnology)

Today, we are surrounded by technology integrated into health in our daily lives, homes, and offices [21]. With the use of technology in healthcare, interdisciplinary products, systems, and treatment options are being developed [6]. Developments in the field of technology have enabled the growth of videoconferencing systems, smartphones, virtual reality, and telehealth services [21].

For technology to be easily used by everyone, it should be accessible, effective, and interesting [6]. It is known that some geriatric individuals are not good at using technology [2]. Worldwide, geriatric individuals have lower levels of access to the Internet than adults, with only 7% of individuals aged 65 years and over connecting to the Internet. In the USA, 44% of geriatric individuals aged 80 years and older are reported to use the Internet [15]. Geriatric individuals are less likely to use technology for health purposes than younger individuals. In particular, it is known that reasons such as education and income levels, accessibility, usability, technical problems, and data management lead to this situation [11]. The benefits and advantages of digital health applications such as telerehabilitation are unequal in all age groups. In particular, due to lower digital literacy in geriatric individuals, the utilization rate of such applications decreases. Reviews show that motivation, accessibility, convenience, and perceived benefits increase the use of digital health applications such as telerehabilitation in geriatric individuals [22].

Due to the differences in the countries' infrastructure, access to the Internet is different. When we look at the European countries in terms of the number of individuals with Internet access problems, it is 32% in Kosovo. In comparison, this rate drops to 1% in Scandinavian countries such as Iceland and Norway [15]. In addition, it is very important to support stakeholders within the health system, such as physiotherapists, geriatric individuals, and carers, in using digital health technologies [9].

Digital health technologies, which include technologies such as e-health, wearable devices, telehealth, and health information technology, offer an accessible, innovative, and comprehensive healthcare service in the field of healthcare. With digital health technologies, medical information can be provided to patients, they can communicate with health professionals, their symptoms and additional diseases can be visualized, and the rehabilitation process can be followed [22].

The term telerehabilitation refers to the delivery of rehabilitation through electronic communication technologies [3]. Telerehabilitation is a method that includes various applications such as therapeutic exercise, imaging, assessment, evaluation, treatment, and education, with or without synchronization, through messaging, web pages, telephone calls, or videoconferencing methods [11]. Telerehabilitation services are provided through various means such as technology, telephone, videoconferencing, chat, or apps [10]. Today, Internet-based remote rehabilitation systems are frequently used as telerehabilitation applications with the help of portable smart devices such as mobile phones and computers [17].

Telerehabilitation via real-time videoconferencing requires basic computer skills and Internet access [15]. The main challenges of telerehabilitation among geriatric individuals are Internet access, lack of familiarity with technology, and digital literacy [1]. Being digitally literate in geriatric patients is one of the enabling conditions for telerehabilitation practices [13]. On the other hand, barriers to the use of digital health services such as telerehabilitation are personal preferences (time, priority, cost) and technical problems in healthy geriatric individuals, while physical and cognitive issues and safety-related concerns in geriatric individuals with chronic and systemic conditions and comorbidities [22]. It has been noted that the security problem can be eliminated with the support of a partner or caregiver in geriatric individuals. The Internet and technology use rate is increasing daily in geriatric individuals and has even increased thrice since 2004 [16].

In conclusion, for telerehabilitation systems to be useful, the Internet and technology usage status of geriatric individuals and their tendency to use innovative rehabilitation approaches may need to be analyzed.

10.4 Telerehabilitation

Although telehealth has been used since the 1940s, it has become more focused in recent years. Telehealth can be described as a broad umbrella encompassing clinical and non-clinical services delivered remotely [18]. Telehealth technologies have an important role in health sciences and medicine in providing remote monitoring and rehabilitation services [23].

The value of the telehealth market is growing every year. The market, approximately 200 billion dollars in 2019, is estimated to reach approximately 400 billion dollars in 2024. Telehealth companies generated revenues of roughly $20 billion in 2020. As technology is integrated into the health sciences, more healthcare startups are entering the digital healthcare market [19]. Telehealth is a remote intervention using electronic communications to protect, promote, and support patients' health

[18]. Telerehabilitation, which includes assessment, diagnosis, and treatment, is one of the specialized areas of telehealth [6]. Telerehabilitation is a sub-branch of telehealth that provides healthcare services to disabled geriatric individuals [7].

Telerehabilitation, a sub-branch of telemedicine, provides remote support, assessment, or some treatment applications to individuals with disabilities via telecommunications [24]. The term telemedicine refers to the provision of remote health system services to patients using communication technologies. Telerehabilitation, a sub-branch of telemedicine applications, can be performed at any patient-determined period [14]. Telerehabilitation, one of the important components of telemedicine and e-health, has developed rapidly in recent years and has been accepted by many people [1]. The American Physical Therapy Association supports telehealth applications to reduce costs and eliminate inequality in healthcare [25].

Current advances in medical and technological sciences are changing how healthcare services are provided to geriatric individuals while extending the human life span [6]. With the help of medicine and technology, rapid developments in Internet technology have enabled the production of a platform that allows rehabilitation practices to be provided remotely to avoid disrupting health systems during the pandemic [17]. Telerehabilitation is a telecommunication-based application platform designed to provide healthcare services to patients or clients in clinical centers or home care services [1]. Telerehabilitation is a system for providing remote healthcare services to patients needing rehabilitation [7]. The decrease in face-to-face treatment options and the rapid spread of the coronavirus have increased the acceptance of telerehabilitation by patients, especially geriatric individuals [6]. Telerehabilitation practices initiated during the COVID-19 pandemic may provide benefits, especially for those far from the clinical center who have limited access to transportation or are concerned about going out in public and the risk of transmission [11].

The delivery of rehabilitation practices in patients' homes through telecommunication networks is called telerehabilitation [20]. Telerehabilitation refers to the remote delivery of different healthcare applications, such as occupational therapy, physiotherapy, speech therapy, and telemonitoring of patients through telecommunication technology [17]. Telerehabilitation is defined as delivering remote rehabilitation services to patients through information and communication technologies by healthcare professionals regardless of time and place [16].

The platform provided with the help of information technologies that include many health services such as assessment, monitoring, prevention, interventions, education, and counseling is called telerehabilitation [26]. With telerehabilitation, also known as virtual physiotherapy [25], physiotherapists can simultaneously provide rehabilitation services to many patients at home, no matter how far away they are from the patients [23]. Telerehabilitation enables many interventions to be performed remotely [6]. In this way, physiotherapists can design a patient-specific, long-term, and comprehensive rehabilitation program for their patients [23].

Increased awareness of different learning styles and the emergence of new technologies have enabled a wide range of telerehabilitation methods to be applied [10].

The main purpose of telerehabilitation is to provide rehabilitation applications at home to patients who cannot go to a hospital/clinical center due to disability level or distance [20]. Telerehabilitation, which has an interactive interface and provides access to information, can include therapeutic interventions, disease management, care services, education of caregivers, and multidisciplinary access to different health professionals [1].

Telerehabilitation is a field where the focus of treatment is on rehabilitation for individuals with cognitive, biopsychosocial, and physical impairments [6]. Since telerehabilitation is a current method that aims to improve patients' motor, mental, or psychological disabilities [14], it is particularly advantageous for geriatric individuals.

During the coronavirus pandemic, many healthcare professionals, especially physiotherapists, made a forced transition from face-to-face treatment to telerehabilitation [11]. The COVID-19 pandemic 2019 has increased emphasis on telemedicine and telerehabilitation worldwide [25]. The COVID-19 pandemic has increased the use of telehealth systems services, especially telerehabilitation [19]. Therefore, the possible use, appropriateness, and accessibility of telerehabilitation applications, especially in geriatric individuals, have increased and accelerated due to epidemics such as COVID-19 [12].

10.5 Advantages and Disadvantages of Telerehabilitation in Geriatrics

There are some advantages of using telemedicine applications in community-based rehabilitation. The first advantage is that if videoconferencing systems are installed in community centers, patients will have easier access to health services. The second advantage is that it promotes learning in group exercise sessions. The last advantage is that it allows real-time interaction between patients and health professionals [24]. By implementing comprehensive treatment options for chronic diseases and disabilities at home through remote monitoring, hospital stays of geriatric individuals can be reduced, and health expenditures can be reduced. Telerehabilitation applications can contribute to these problems [7]. Telerehabilitation can reduce functional capacity deficits in geriatric individuals [13]. Moreover, data from around the world report that advanced age alone is not a barrier to using telerehabilitation [16]. In addition, in 2019, more than 50% of the world's population had access to the Internet [15]. Despite all this, unfortunately, telerehabilitation is often considered a plan B for geriatric individuals [13].

Telerehabilitation is increasingly used for many reasons, including reduced travel time, easy access to specialists in rural areas, continuity of care, and reduced costs [21]. The potential benefits of telerehabilitation in geriatrics are presented in Fig. 10.1 [6].

Telerehabilitation can be easily applied after the acute phase in non-clinical settings. For example, with telerehabilitation, the continuation of rehabilitation in the hospital can be used in the community or at home. In addition, telerehabilitation can

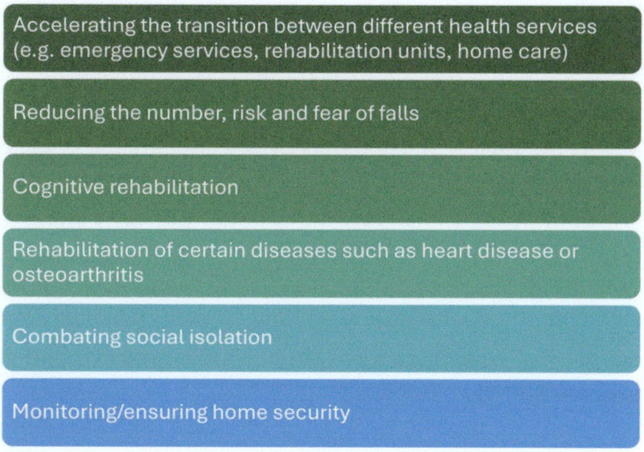

Fig. 10.1 Potential benefits of telerehabilitation in geriatrics

improve the functionality of patients and reduce long-term disability and healthcare costs [24]. Telerehabilitation, which can potentially manage many components of health, including patients' level of functional independence, self-care, and disease management, can also improve traditional home care [7]. One advantage of telerehabilitation is facilitating the transition to home care after discharge [6].

In the USA, patients who want to receive 20 min of face-to-face healthcare from healthcare professionals spend an average of 2 h for travel and waiting time during this visit [6]. Telerehabilitation practices are more advantageous for patients who live in areas far from the hospital or clinical center or who have physical disabilities [14]. The main advantages of telerehabilitation include less transportation and transportation costs, and more time for the healthcare professional to spend with the patient. Telerehabilitation is an alternative treatment method for geriatric individuals who have multiple diseases and have difficulty in going to hospitals or clinical centers [6]. Telerehabilitation applications can protect geriatric patients from infections that are common in the hospital environment or provide geriatric patients who live far from the clinical center with the treatment option they need [3].

In conclusion, a telerehabilitation service can be beneficial for both patients and healthcare professionals [6].

Despite all these advantages of telerehabilitation, various security issues, lack of digital literacy, and age-related conditions may negatively affect the spread of telerehabilitation among geriatric individuals [16]. Telerehabilitation via real-time videoconferencing requires basic computer skills and Internet access [15]. In addition, the disadvantages of telerehabilitation include the limitation of clinical physical examination, administrative barriers, and technical problems such as identification and data security [21].

Telerehabilitation may be a more cost-effective treatment option than home-based or center-based rehabilitation. However, it may be more difficult for geriatric individuals to benefit from therapeutic exercises through telerehabilitation. The main reason for this is that close supervision may be required to ensure that exercises are performed correctly and properly for geriatric individuals, who are a group that may experience more health problems [11]. Furthermore, it should not be overlooked that inequalities may occur in the healthcare system if telerehabilitation practices are not explained to the geriatric population in a detailed and accessible way [6].

In conclusion, despite the current advantages of technology and the rapid adaptation of healthcare professionals to telerehabilitation, there is a need for basic protocol definitions (to whom, by whom, and how treatment will be administered) in telerehabilitation [6]. In addition, access to telerehabilitation services may be limited due to geriatric patients' and caregivers' concerns about telerehabilitation practices, data privacy, Internet connectivity, legal barriers, insurance issues, cultural adaptation, language problems, and cognitive, biopsychosocial, and behavioral problems [12].

10.6 Examples of Telerehabilitation Usage in Geriatrics

Telerehabilitation is a newly introduced method whose effects have been investigated in recent years [26]. The increasing popularity and prevalence of the telerehabilitation option among clinicians and patients offers researchers the opportunity to examine the effectiveness of this method and publish its results [6].

The number of studies investigating the effectiveness of telerehabilitation in the literature is increasing daily. The effects of telerehabilitation have been investigated in patients with Parkinson's disease, heart attack, stroke, and surgery [3]. The impacts of telerehabilitation in patients with spinal cord injuries, multiple sclerosis, hemiplegia, orthopedic or brain traumas, and pressure ulcers have been examined, and studies showing that it is beneficial have been published in the literature [24]. The results of studies investigating the effects of telerehabilitation in different diseases and conditions are encouraging and promising [9]. Telerehabilitation is mostly applied in treating heart and lung diseases [14]. While many studies in the literature examine the effects of telerehabilitation on neurological, musculoskeletal, oncological, and cardiopulmonary pathologies, the number of studies focusing on the geriatric population is limited [16].

Telerehabilitation seems to be one of the ideal applications for geriatric patients due to their poor physical condition [14]. Telerehabilitation is an important method to increase or maintain the level of independence of geriatric patients at home and to prevent hospitalization of geriatric patients [26]. Telerehabilitation has been reported to be a promising method for implementing geriatric rehabilitation [9]. It is unknown whether the exercise-based telerehabilitation method provided through synchronized videoconferencing is as effective as conventional physiotherapy for geriatric individuals [11].

Since telerehabilitation allows rehabilitation from home, includes caregiver or family participation in rehabilitation, and avoids travel obstacles, the effectiveness of telerehabilitation in neurological patients with movement disorders such as spinal cord injury, multiple sclerosis, amyotrophic lateral sclerosis has been examined, and high satisfaction of the patients has been encountered [21]. It has been reported in studies that the level of pain and disability in patients with chronic neck pain decreases with telerehabilitation. It has also been indicated that telerehabilitation improves functionality in patients with Parkinson's disease, stroke, cardiopulmonary and oncologic diseases. It has been noted that telerehabilitation provides functional improvements during walking, transfer tasks, and activities of daily living in geriatric patients [25].

Telerehabilitation is used to improve the long-term effectiveness of treatment [10]. It has been reported that telerehabilitation performed in groups via videoconferencing yielded similar results compared to a traditional exercise program with supervised supervision. Although it is unlikely that telerehabilitation can be applied to geriatric inpatients, telerehabilitation can be successfully applied to many patients with different diagnoses [13]. Studies also show that telerehabilitation with a high level of compliance with home programs is similar to or even better than face-to-face treatments in terms of clinical outcomes [10]. In another study, telerehabilitation applied as rehabilitation was reported to be effective on patient outcomes [23].

Home-based telerehabilitation was compared with traditional rehabilitation practices in geriatric patients undergoing total knee arthroplasty surgery. In this randomized controlled trial, 21 patients (66 ± 10 years) who had undergone arthroplasty received a home-based physiotherapy program in telerehabilitation for 2 months, two sessions per week for 16 sessions. The physiotherapy approaches applied in the treatment program were based on increasing the functionality of the patient's daily living activities. The study compared a range of motion values, balance and muscle strength levels, and knee functionality scores in patients who received home-based telerehabilitation and those treated with the traditional approach. It was reported that there were significant improvements in all parameters in both groups at the end of 8 weeks, and it was found that neither group was superior to the other [27].

In a total of 112 geriatric patients with chronic obstructive pulmonary disease and chronic heart failure, home-based telerehabilitation was compared with a standard care program, including medical care, oxygen support, and general practitioner visits. In the randomized controlled trial, 56 geriatric patients received a personalized home-based telerehabilitation program by a physiotherapist for 4 months. The home-based telerehabilitation program was implemented at a basic and advanced level. The basic level telerehabilitation program included 15–25 min of mini-ergometer exercise, 30 min of calisthenic exercises, and free walking. The advanced telerehabilitation program included 30–45 min of mini-ergometer exercise with increasing load, 30–45 min of muscle strengthening exercises, and walking for 3–7 days. Aerobic capacity, dyspnea and disability levels, physical activity, and quality of life scores of the geriatric patients participating in the study were evaluated by the 6-Minute Walk Test, Medical Research Council, Barthel Index, Physical Activity Profile, and Minnesota Living with Heart Failure Questionnaire or COPD Assessment Test, respectively. After 4 months, it was reported that the home-based telerehabilitation program showed statistically greater improvements in disease-specific outcomes compared to the standard care program [28].

Wu et al. investigated the effects of telerehabilitation for 6 months in geriatric patients undergoing total hip arthroplasty following hip fracture. In the study, 85 geriatric patients were randomly divided into two different groups. One group received a home-based telerehabilitation program, while the other received a telephone follow-up. In the telephone follow-up group, patients were advised to follow the exercise program recommended by the physiotherapist, and regular telephone contact was established. Geriatric patients in the telerehabilitation group were asked to regularly watch and then perform the therapeutic exercise videos personalized by the physiotherapist, which included information on balance and cardiopulmonary exercises, self-care, and activities of daily living. Harris hip scores, functional independence levels, and anxiety scores of the geriatric patients included in the study were evaluated 1, 3, and 6 months after surgery. In addition, postoperative complications were reported. As a result of the study, compared to the telephone group, geriatric patients in the telerehabilitation group showed significantly better improvements in Harris hip scores, functional independence, and anxiety levels at 1, 3, and 6 months. In addition, geriatric patients in the telerehabilitation group had significantly lower complication rates than those in the telephone group [14].

Finally, a systematic review examining telerehabilitation's effectiveness in assisting the geriatric population during the COVID-19 pandemic included 2529 articles in the initial search. The study reported that telerehabilitation had similar or sometimes even more effective outcomes compared to conventional and standard treatments. Therefore, it was concluded that telerehabilitation may be a complementary option to traditional therapies in geriatrics, especially during pandemic periods [12].

10.7 Conclusion

Telerehabilitation and its spread among the population depend primarily on healthcare professionals [18]. The more healthcare professionals use, investigate, and examine the effects of current and innovative methods, such as telerehabilitation, on geriatric patients, the more evidence-based knowledge will develop and clarify. The number of studies examining the effects of telerehabilitation in geriatric individuals is increasing day by day. Although it has been shown that telerehabilitation positively contributes to geriatric individuals with different diseases, it is thought too early to be accepted as a method to be applied as a first choice in every disease. In conclusion, in light of all this information, it is suggested that telerehabilitation may be a potential option for geriatric individuals since it shows promising and encouraging results.

References

1. Md Fadzil NH, Shahar S, Rajikan R, Singh DKA, Mat Ludin AF, Subramaniam P, Ibrahim N, Vanoh D, Mohamad AN. A scoping review for usage of telerehabilitation among older adults with mild cognitive impairment or cognitive frailty. Int J Environ Res Public Health. 2022;19(7):4000.
2. Chaves Filho AC, Inocêncio AV, Ferreira KR, Cavalcante EL, Bispo BC, Rodrigues CM, Lessa PS, Rodrigues MA. Geriatric physiotherapy: a telerehabilitation system for identifying therapeutic exercises. In: Brazilian Congress on Biomedical Engineering. Cham: Springer International Publishing; 2020. p. 969–74.
3. Fakontis C, Iakovidis P, Lytras D, Kasimis K, Kottaras A, Chasapis G. The efficacy of telerehabilitation in older adults after a hip injury: a narrative review. Crit Rev Phys Rehabil Med. 2022;34(1):17–28.
4. Saito T, Izawa KP. Effectiveness and feasibility of home-based telerehabilitation for community-dwelling elderly people in Southeast Asian countries and regions: a systematic review. Aging Clin Exp Res. 2021;33(10):2657–69.
5. Groom LL, McCarthy MM, Stimpfel AW, Brody AA. Telemedicine and telehealth in nursing homes: an integrative review. J Am Med Dir Assoc. 2021;22(9):1784–1801.e7.
6. Oh-Park M, Lew HL, Raghavan P. Telerehabilitation for geriatrics. Phys Med Rehabil Clin. 2021;32(2):291–305.
7. Bendixen RM, Levy CE, Olive ES, Kobb RF, Mann WC. Cost effectiveness of a telerehabilitation program to support chronically ill and disabled elders in their homes. Telemed J E Health. 2009;15(1):31–8.
8. Bendixen RM, Horn K, Levy C. Using telerehabilitation to support elders with chronic illness in their homes. Top Geriatr Rehabil. 2007;23(1):47–51.
9. Pol M, Qadeer A, van Hartingsveldt M, Choukou MA. Perspectives of rehabilitation professionals on implementing a validated home telerehabilitation intervention for older adults in geriatric rehabilitation: multisite focus group study. JMIR Rehabil Assist Technol. 2023;10:e44498.
10. Jirasakulsuk N, Saengpromma P, Khruakhorn S. Real-time telerehabilitation in older adults with musculoskeletal conditions: systematic review and meta-analysis. JMIR Rehabil Assist Technol. 2022;9(3):e36028.
11. Wicks M, Dennett AM, Peiris CL. Physiotherapist-led, exercise-based telerehabilitation for older adults improves patient and health service outcomes: a systematic review and meta-analysis. Age Ageing. 2023;52(11):afad207.
12. Ahmadi Marzaleh M, Peyravi M, Azhdari N, Bahaadinbeigy K, Sarpourian F. Application of telerehabilitation for older adults during the COVID-19 pandemic: a systematic review. Disaster Med Public Health Prep. 2022;17:e402.
13. Jørgensen BB, Gregersen M, Pallesen SH, Marie DE. Tele-rehabilitation in community-dwelling older people with reduced functional capacity: a 4-patient case report. Gerontol Geriatr Med. 2022;8:23337214221109820.
14. Wu WY, Zhang YG, Zhang YY, Peng B, Xu WG. Clinical effectiveness of home-based telerehabilitation program for geriatric hip fracture following total hip replacement. Orthop Surg. 2023;15(2):423–31.
15. Jørgensen BB, Gregersen M, Pallesen SH, Damsgaard EM. A group-based real-time videoconferencing telerehabilitation programme in recently discharged geriatric patients: a feasibility study. Eur Geriatr Med. 2021;12(4):801–8.
16. Gamble CJ, van Haastregt J, van Dam van Isselt EF, Zwakhalen S, Schols J. Effectiveness of guided telerehabilitation on functional performance in community dwelling older adults: a systematic review. Clin Rehabil. 2024;38(4):457–77.
17. Zhang YY, Zhang YG, Li Z, Li SH, Xu WG. Effect of home-based telerehabilitation on the postoperative rehabilitation outcome of hip fracture in the aging population. Orthop Surg. 2022;14(8):1768–77.

18. Jaswal S, Lo J, Sithamparanathan G, Nowrouzi-Kia B. The era of technology in healthcare: an evaluation of telerehabilitation on patient outcomes-a systematic review and meta-analysis protocol. Syst Rev. 2023;12(1):76.
19. Chakraborty I, Edirippulige S, Vigneswara Ilavarasan P. The role of telehealth startups in healthcare service delivery: a systematic review. Int J Med Inform. 2023;174:105048.
20. Hamel M, Fontaine R, Boissy P. In-home telerehabilitation for geriatric patients. IEEE Eng Med Biol Mag. 2008;27(4):29–37.
21. Matsumoto ME, Wilske GC, Tapia R. Innovative approaches to delivering telehealth. Phys Med Rehabil Clin N Am. 2021;32(2):451–65.
22. Hasnan S, Aggarwal S, Mohammadi L, Koczwara B. Barriers and enablers of uptake and adherence to digital health interventions in older patients with cancer: a systematic review. J Geriatr Oncol. 2022;13(8):1084–91.
23. De Souza Miguel GF, de Sá AA, de Souza JT, Naves EL. Home-based telerehabilitation: a review of remote therapy frameworks. Res Soc Dev. 2021;10(6):e4910615489.
24. Lai JC, Woo J, Hui E, Chan WM. Telerehabilitation—a new model for community-based stroke rehabilitation. J Telemed Telecare. 2004;10(4):199–205.
25. Havran MA, Bidelspach DE. Virtual physical therapy and telerehabilitation. Phys Med Rehabil Clin N Am. 2021;32(2):419–28.
26. Reeder B, Chung J, Stevens-Lapsley J. Current telerehabilitation research with older adults at home: an integrative review. J Gerontol Nurs. 2016;42(10):15–20.
27. Tousignant M, Moffet H, Boissy P, Corriveau H, Cabana F, Marquis F. A randomized controlled trial of home telerehabilitation for post-knee arthroplasty. J Telemed Telecare. 2011;17(4):195–8.
28. Bernocchi P, Vitacca M, La Rovere MT, Volterrani M, Galli T, Baratti D, Paneroni M, Campolongo G, Sposato B, Scalvini S. Home-based telerehabilitation in older patients with chronic obstructive pulmonary disease and heart failure: a randomised controlled trial. Age Ageing. 2018;47(1):82–8.

Ethics in Teleassessment

11

Mehmet Gürhan Karakaya and İlkim Çıtak Karakaya

11.1 Teleassessment

11.1.1 Definition, Types, and Tools of Teleassessment

Teleassessment refers to the remote assessment of patients by health professionals using digital technologies such as computers, tablets, or smartphones [1]. Teleassessment methods can be analyzed in two sections: synchronous (simultaneous) and asynchronous methods (see Fig. 11.1) [2, 3].

Clinicians can use simple equipment and more advanced methods requiring web-based systems or virtual reality-based formats while assessing patients in remote areas. Methods that can be used as a teleassessment tool are:

- Mobile application(s)
- Videoconferences
  - Zoom, Skype, Teams, WhatsApp, etc.
- Telephone conferences
- Environment (camera) sensors
  - Motion capture systems, infrared camera sensor (Kinect etc.)
- Wearable sensors
  - Physical activity monitoring, Inertial Measurement Unit (IMU), Pressure, Surface (sEMG, sEEG, sECG)
- Virtual reality
- Tele-robots
- Artificial intelligence [2–6]

M. G. Karakaya (✉) · İ. Çıtak Karakaya
Department of Physiotherapy and Rehabilitation, Faculty of Health Sciences, Muğla Sıtkı Koçman University, Muğla, Türkiye
e-mail: mgkarakaya@mu.edu.tr

F. Özden et al. (eds.), *Telerehabilitation*, TELe-Health,
https://doi.org/10.1007/978-3-031-69080-8_11

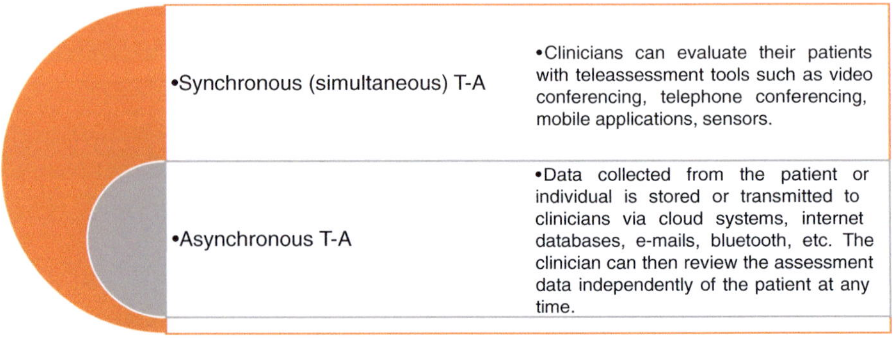

Fig. 11.1 Synchronous and asynchronous teleassessment

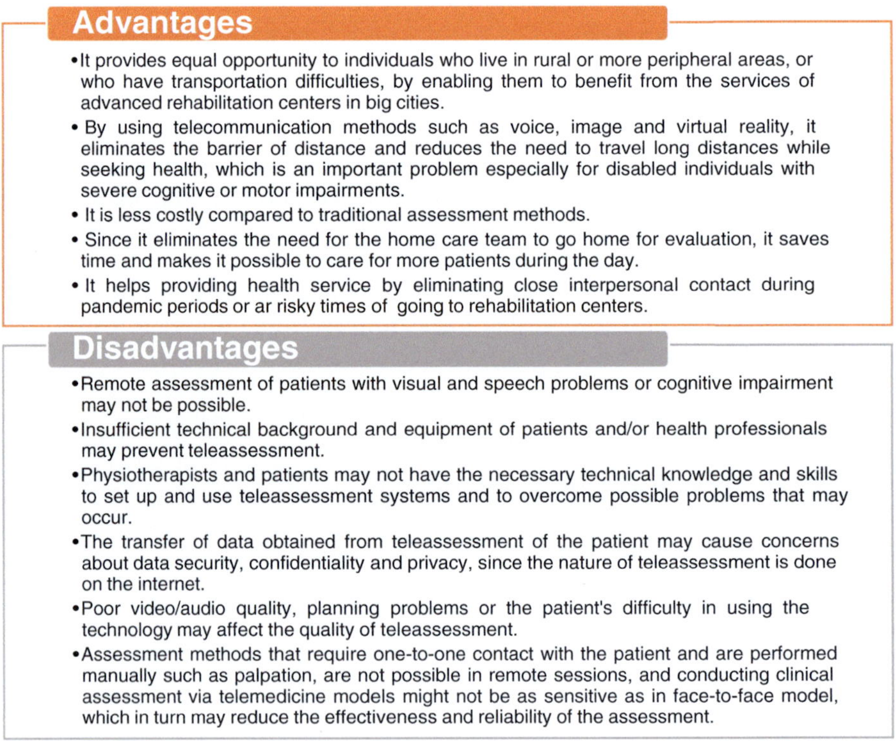

Fig. 11.2 Advantages and disadvantages of teleassessment

11.1.2 Advantages and Disadvantages of Teleassessment

The advantages and disadvantages of teleassessment applications can be stated as in Fig. 11.2 [3–5, 7–9]:

11.1.3 Validity and Reliability of Teleassessments

Randomized controlled trials, systematic reviews and/or meta-analyses are available that investigate whether teleassessments are valid and reliable compared to traditional face-to-face assessments [4]. Teleassessment as a tool to determine functional capacity and lower limb performance is feasible and valid compared to face-to-face assessment in healthy individuals [10]. In systematic reviews conducted to investigate the reliability and validity of teleassessment methods in patients with musculoskeletal problems, concurrent validity was found to be high for pain, edema, range of motion, muscle strength, balance, and gait evaluations; intermediate for special orthopedic tests (SOT) and neurodynamic tests (NDT); and low for lumbar spine posture assessment. However, inter-rater and intra-rater reliability were reported as good or excellent [4, 11]. In a study conducted in neurological patient groups, test-retest reliability of teleassessments for balance, gait, and motor function was found to be good in acute stroke patients and excellent in chronic stroke patients. It was reported that asynchronous and synchronous teleassessment methods had excellent reliability and validity in chronic stroke patients, eliminating the need for a therapist to be present during the test [12].

11.2 Ethical Issues in Teleassessment

Due to the holistic nature of the rehabilitation concept, rehabilitation assessments include comprehensive examinations and evaluations to understand the individual's situation and develop an intervention plan that best suits their needs. Therefore, these assessments include the biological, physiological, and functional states of individuals and their psychological and social states [13]. Teleassessments are made by a wide range of rehabilitation professionals such as physical therapists, speech-language pathologists, occupational therapists, audiologists, rehabilitation physicians, nurses, psychologists, and dietitians; therefore, as with face-to-face practices, all professional team members need clear guidelines for acting ethically during both teleassessments and telerehabilitation approaches. The lack of international standards and applicable legal provisions is one of the biggest obstacles to these applications' effective and widespread use. Developing such standards is quite difficult due to the broad content of telerehabilitation, the professional diversity of its practitioners, and the fact that these professions have different autonomy due to the legal regulations in the countries where they practice [13, 14]. In some countries and regions, religious and cultural implications are of high value in delivering the health system [4, 13]. For this reason, the ethical principles to be followed in telerehabilitation assessment and practices should be in line with international standards and determined by considering local needs.

The main ethical issues of teleassessment in rehabilitation may be subtitled as privacy and confidentiality, informed consent, intersectionality, patient-clinician relationship, quality of assessment, data security, and cost-effectiveness. These issues should all be considered based on the basic ethical principles of respect for persons, beneficence, nonmaleficence, and justice [15].

There are no clear ethical guidelines regarding physiotherapy and rehabilitation services via telehealth systems in Turkey. Therefore, this chapter aims to review the ethical issues to be considered, especially by the physiotherapists and by other professional members of the rehabilitation team during teleassessments, and is prepared based on the Regulation on the Provision of Distance Health Services published by the Ministry of Health of the Republic of Türkiye in 2022 [16], and Ethical Principles for Turkish Physiotherapists, published by the Turkish Physiotherapists Association in 2018 [17]. Also, relevant principles and guidelines by national and international authorities related to different fields of rehabilitation, such as the Turkish Psychological Counseling and Guidance Association, the Turkish Psychologist Association, Australian Physiotherapy Association, Chartered Society of Physiotherapy (UK), American Speech-Language-Hearing Association, The Ontario Psychological Association and the Canadian Association of Psychologists in Disability Assessment, Australian Physiotherapy Association helped cover the topic comprehensively [4, 13, 18–20].

11.2.1 Evaluation of Suitability for Teleassessment

A case-by-case professional judgment based on the current condition and capacity of the patient/individual, and willingness and preferences of both the patient/individual and/or the caregiver; available resources and technology; the urgency of medical care; risks and benefits should be made to determine whether teleassessment is appropriate [18, 19, 21]. A direct physical examination, including hands-on assessment, may be required to determine a physiotherapy diagnosis and treatment plan [13, 21]. As reported by Zischke et al. (2021) in a systematic review on the utility of physiotherapy assessments delivered by telehealth, performing specific types of physiotherapy assessments via synchronous forms of telehealth appears to be valid and reliable [4]. These assessment types include range of movement, muscle strength, endurance, pain, special orthopedic tests (shoulder/elbow), Berg Balance Scale, timed up and go, timed stance test, six-minute walk test, steps in 360-degree turn, *Movement Assessment Battery for Children* (2nd Edition), step test, ABILHAND assessment, active straight leg raise, and circumferential measures of the upper limb. They have also stated that the assessment types which are more observational in nature can be performed more easily and have higher levels of validity and reliability [4]. However, in another systematic review on digital vs. conventional face-to-face physiotherapy assessment of patients with musculoskeletal disorders, Bernhardsson et al. (2023) stated that several of the clinical tests commonly used in physiotherapies, such as muscle strength tests, orthopedic tests, nerve tests, and joint assessment, seem particularly difficult to perform using digital technology [22]. They have reported that extremity ROM assessment and patient reported outcome measures (PROMs) had the highest validity, but posture assessment and clinical observations had the lowest validity [22].

While evaluating the suitability for and performing teleassessments, taking a careful history is vital. Rehabilitation professionals should be knowledgeable and aware of the "red flag" conditions such as acute neurological loss (particularly cauda equina syndrome) in musculoskeletal problems. In case of any "red flag" symptoms, they should consider further investigation, safety-netting, referral (routine or urgent), or emergency hospital admission [23].

11.2.2 Evaluator's Profession in Teleassessment

Professional rehabilitation team members should conduct teleassessments in alignment with the ethical principles and standards of their profession, as well as the relevant regulations of the country where they practice [24]. They should be able to provide evidence of being qualified and competent to undertake whatever service they provide if asked through audit or complaint [18]. Being registered with national professional organizations such as the Turkish Physiotherapists Association for Physiotherapists practicing in Turkey or the American Psychological Association for Psychologists in the United States would be beneficial for them.

11.2.3 Qualification of the Evaluator and Establishing Professional Boundaries

Teleassessments require additional specific knowledge and skills beyond the basic assessment competencies of evaluators who conduct in-person evaluations. The professionals who were not trained in teleassessment during their formal education may need additional specific training in telehealth and teleassessment ethics to be comfortable and competent in administering, evaluating data, and evaluating limitations of the teleassessment used [24].

Establishing and maintaining professional boundaries is another ethical issue during teleassessments. Although it may sometimes be tempting to loosen professional boundaries in the telehealth environment, it is ethically appropriate to dress professionally, reduce distractions, and clearly express expectations from patients [25]. These can help to develop a relationship between the patient and the healthcare practitioner based on mutual trust and respect [26].

11.2.4 Informed Consent

As a part of a healthcare service, teleassessment requires that the individual receiving the service sign a consent form after her/his identity is confirmed. This form, which usually includes detailed information about the aim, content, and provision type of the assessments (i.e., entirely via telehealth or a hybrid of face-to-face and teleassessment), should be in plain language and contain information about [13, 18, 24]:

- Who will be providing the teleassessment service (including information about the qualifications and experiences of the physiotherapist)
- The length of the consultation
- The cost and payment arrangements
- Any potential risks and benefits
- Possible threats to privacy and confidentiality of medical information in this model of assessment
- The overall reliability and validity of teleassessment
- Limitations (not being able to see the client's entire body, not being able to administer certain tests, or performance-based tasks being less precise, etc.) and conditions for discontinuing the process
- The availability of in-person services in the relevant geographical location in case of situational factors associated with teleassessment (Internet problems, disruptions, interruptions, etc.)

It should be ensured that the patient/individual knows and understands the teleassessment process, factors that may impede the assessment, and limitations of the process [24]. The ability to give consent depends on the patient's mental state and decision-making capacity. When necessary, an expert decision maker may be appointed to determine whether the patient can give consent [13]. In case the patient/individual cannot provide consent (underage, incompetent, incapacitated, etc.), an appropriate individual, according to applicable legislation and regulatory requirements, signs the informed consent form [18, 27].

The consent should include information about the type and methods of assessment (videotaping, photographs, online forms, etc.), recording and/or storing the data, transmission of information to other healthcare providers or the patient/individual's family, and possible threats to privacy and confidentiality of medical information in this model of assessment [13, 18, 21].

11.2.5 Intersectionality

To provide health equity in rehabilitation services, it is important to understand the intersectionality concept. It highlights how various aspects of an individual's identity can intersect and interact to create unique experiences of discrimination, advantage or disadvantage, or privilege [28]. By considering intersectionality, evaluators should be mindful of the needs of the patients/individuals, put an effort to offer an accessible teleassessment, and avoid using contraindicated/inappropriate assessment methods (i.e., teleassessments that require fine motor proficiency to set up for a patient with motor impairments) [24].

11.2.6 Privacy and Confidentiality

Traditional medicine requires an ethical health relationship based on an unwritten "contract of trust" between the patient and a health professional with special skills and knowledge to heal them. Each health professional is committed by their professional oath to know, respect, and defend the rights of their patients. As new technologies and new telehealth models continue to emerge, the fundamental ethical responsibilities of healthcare professionals remain unchanged. Healthcare professionals should always consider prioritizing patient welfare over other interests, respecting patient privacy and confidentiality, and carrying out a transparent information process while making clinical decisions and using resources both face-to-face and telehealth tools [29, 30].

While the correct meaning and definition of "privacy" is a matter of disagreement in the literature, it is related to the control one has over access to oneself (both physical access and access to information about him/her) [31]. Privacy interests of individuals are not limited to their bodies and personal information but also include expressed thoughts and opinions, personal communications with others, and spaces they occupy [32].

Not only the information related to the observational and clinical assessments but also the perceptions about the patient's lifestyle, family life, and habits are private information. So, inappropriate disclosure of that information may threaten the patient's reputation, opportunities, and human dignity [29]. Therefore, respecting confidentiality and protecting this information is essential to prevent unauthorized access, use, and dissemination.

During teleassessments with both live-interactive and store-and-forward interactions, unauthorized viewing or disclosure may occur, even often quite innocent [29]. To prevent this, professionals shall determine requirements for documentation, storage, and retrieval of client records, and personal and technological safeguards such as secure encrypted systems should be used by the patient and the healthcare professional [19, 29]. Limiting the availability of information to those people who need to know (other health professionals, family members, caregivers, etc.) is required [19]. It should be kept in mind that during teleassessment, it can be challenging to maintain privacy due to poor socioeconomics and complex family dynamics (i.e., many family members attending the teleassessment session due to inadequate residence conditions or to cultural/religious backgrounds) [13]. For instance, teleassessments that require the patient to be undressed in front of a camera may be considered as a privacy problem by the patient and/or the family member attending the session.

11.2.7 Data Collection and Protection

During teleassessments, health professionals should do their best with what they have available to them, as long as what they are doing is mindful and ethical. Teleassessment management procedures should be as close as possible to traditional management, with attempts to adapt procedures to mimic what is experienced in a face-to-face administration [33].

A safety protocol should be planned in advance to be in place in case of an emergency or adverse event (heart attack, fall, etc.). Alternative methods for contacting the patient (e.g., telephone) should also be established to be used in case of an Internet failure. It would be good to test all technologies before patient appointments to ensure the good functioning of the teleassessment system [21].

Health professionals should be rigorously mindful of the quality of the data collected. To do this, they should remain vigilant about what is occurring on the patient's side and need to remain focused on potential distractors and interruptions and adapt their procedures accordingly [33].

All devices used for teleassessments must be registered and licensed with the relevant party, such as the ministries of the countries [13]. Not only the ones who supply the device but also the health professionals are responsible for the maintenance, use, and replacement of devices [34].

Telerehabilitation professionals use various data collection tools during remote assessments, which require specific qualifications such as professional license and certification or permissions for those protected by copyright laws [24, 34].

For software applications to be used in remote physiotherapy and rehabilitation evaluations and for non-open access, licensed and/or paid evaluation methods such as some self-report outcome measures, permission must be obtained, and copyright must not be violated. Test security should not be undermined, and it should be remembered that it is easier for patients/individuals to take screenshots of materials presented on their own devices and copy printed materials sent out to them. Therefore, telerehabilitation professionals need to be clear with their patients about what is and is not allowed for these materials used when conducting teleassessments and collecting data [13, 24, 33, 34].

The evaluators who conduct teleassessments are responsible to take steps to protect data security. They should consider using password protections, encryption, and malware protection and keeping backups to store the paper protocols and electronic forms securely. All steps taken for data security should be documented and stated in the evaluation report [25, 33, 34].

References

1. Karakaya MG. Ergoterapide Teknoloji Temelli Aktiviteler. In: Yücel H, editor. Aktivite Temelli Ergoterapi. 1st ed. Ankara: Hipokrat Yayıncılık; 2020. p. 523–49.
2. Vaikuntharajan P, Tobis M, Richardson J. Telephone-delivered physiotherapy interventions improve physical function for adults with a chronic condition: a systematic review and meta-analysis. Arch Phys Med Rehabil. 2022;103(1):131–44. e14. https://doi.org/10.1016/j.apmr.2021.05.022.
3. Karakaya MG, Ercan Yüceer Ş. Fizyoterapi ve Rehabilitasyonda Teledeğerlendirme. In: Ki KN, Kayabınar E, Türkmen C, editors. Telerehabilitasyon, Fizyoterapi Uygulamaları. Ankara: Hipokrat Yayıncılık; 2022. p. 19–34.

4. Zischke C, Simas V, Hing W, Milne N, Spittle A, Pope R. The utility of physiotherapy assessments delivered by telehealth: a systematic review. J Glob Health. 2021;11:04072. https://doi.org/10.7189/jogh.11.04072.
5. Karakaya MG, Murat G. İnme Tanılı Hastalarda Telerehabilitasyon. In: Ki KN, Kayabınar E, Türkmen C, editors. Telerehabilitasyon, Fizyoterapi Uygulamaları. Ankara: Hipokrat Yayıncılık; 2022. p. 141–56.
6. Karakaya MG, Çıtak Karakaya İ, Aksu YS. İnme Rehabilitasyonunda Teknolojinin Kullanımı. In: Karaduman A, Aksu Yıldırım S, Tunca Yılmaz Ö, editors. İnme Sonrası Fizyoterapi ve Rehabilitasyon. Ankara: Hipokrat Kitapevi; 2016. p. 173–89.
7. Hailey D, Roine R, Ohinmaa A, Dennett L. Evidence of benefit from telerehabilitation in routine care: a systematic review. J Telemed Telecare. 2011;17(6):281–7.
8. Torsney K. Advantages and disadvantages of telerehabilitation for persons with neurological disabilities. NeuroRehabilitation. 2003;18(2):183–5.
9. Russell TG. Telerehabilitation: a coming of age. Aust J Physiother. 2009;55(1):5–6.
10. Mavronasou A, Asimakos A, Vasilopoulos A, Katsaounou P, Kortianou EA. Remote administration of the short physical performance battery, the 1-minute sit to stand, and the Chester step test in post-COVID-19 patients after hospitalization: establishing inter-reliability and agreement with the face-to-face assessment. Disabil Rehabil. 2023:1–11. https://doi.org/10.1080/09638288.2023.2297928.
11. Mani S, Sharma S, Omar B, Paungmali A, Joseph L. Validity and reliability of Internet-based physiotherapy assessment for musculoskeletal disorders: a systematic review. J Telemed Telecare. 2017;23(3):379–91.
12. Önal B, Köse N, Önal ŞN, Zengin HY. Validity and intra-and inter-rater reliability of the Tinetti performance-oriented mobility assessment balance subscale using different tele-assessment methods in patients with chronic stroke. Top Stroke Rehabil. 2024;31:547–55.
13. Alhabter AM, Qureshi AZ, Ullah S. Ethical and legal aspects of telerehabilitation in Saudi Arabia. Int J Telerehabil. 2023;15(2):e6569. https://doi.org/10.5195/ijt.2023.6569.
14. Özden F, Lembraki Y. The ethical necessities and principles in telerehabilitation. Sağlık Hizmetleri ve Eğitimi Dergisi. 2020;3(2):35–7.
15. Clark PA, Capuzzi K, Harrison J. Telemedicine: medical, legal and ethical perspectives. Med Sci Monit. 2010;16(12):RA261–72.
16. Ministry of Health of the Republic of Türkiye. Uzaktan Sağlık Hizmetlerinin Sunumu Hakkında Yönetmelik. TC Resmi Gazete. 10 Feb 2022. Number: 31746.
17. Turkish Physiotherapists Association. Ethical principles for Turkish physiotherapists. 21 Oct 2018. https://www.fizyoterapistler.org.tr/etik-prensipler. Accessed 17 Apr 2024.
18. Australian Physiotherapy Association. Telehealth guidelines response to COVID-19. Mar 2020. https://australian.physio/sites/default/files/APATelehealthGuidelinesCOVID190420FA.pdf. Accessed 17 Apr 2024.
19. Brennan D, Tindall L, Theodoros D, Brown J, Campbell M, Christiana D, et al. A blueprint for telerehabilitation guidelines. Int J Telerehabil. 2010;2(2):31–4. https://doi.org/10.5195/ijt.2010.6063.
20. American Speech-Language-Hearing Association. Code of ethics. 1 Mar 2023. https://www.asha.org/policy/et2016-00342/. Accessed 17 Apr 2024.
21. College of Physical Therapists of British Columbia. Telerehabilitation guide. Apr 2024. https://cptbc.org/wp-content/uploads/2024/04/CPTBC_Telerehabilitation-Guide_April2_2024.pdf. Accessed 17 Apr 2024.
22. Bernhardsson S, Larsson A, Bergenheim A, Ho-Henriksson CM, Ekhammar A, Lange E, et al. Digital physiotherapy assessment vs conventional face-to-face physiotherapy assessment of patients with musculoskeletal disorders: a systematic review. PLoS One. 2023;18(3):e0283013. https://doi.org/10.1371/journal.pone.0283013.
23. Murray T, Murray G, Murray J. Remote musculoskeletal assessment framework: a guide for primary care. Cureus. 2021;13(1):e12778. https://doi.org/10.7759/cureus.12778.

24. Educational Testing Service-ETS. Tele-assessment guidance for psychological, psychoeducational and neuropsychological assessment. 2023. https://www.ets.org/pdfs/disabilities/tele-assessment-guidance.pdf. Accessed 18 Apr 2024.
25. Psychological Assessment Products-PAR. Ten ethical teleassessment considerations for practitioners. 26 July 2022. https://blog.parinc.com/ten-ethical-teleassessment-considerations-for-practitioners. Accessed 18 Apr 2024.
26. Health Professions Council of South Africa. General ethical guidelines for good practice in telehealth. Dec 2021. https://www.hpcsa.co.za/Uploads/professional_practice/ethics/Booklet_10_Telehealth_Dec_2021_v2.pdf. Accessed 18 Apr 2024.
27. College of Physical Therapists of British Columbia. Informed consent. 4 Mar 2024. https://cptbc.org/wp-content/uploads/2024/03/CPTBC_Standards_2024_InformedConsent.pdf. Accessed 18 Apr 2024.
28. Quigley A, Myezwa H, McArthur C. Editorial: equity, diversity, and inclusion in rehabilitation sciences. Front Rehabil Sci. 2023;4:1334054. https://doi.org/10.3389/fresc.2023.1334054.
29. Fleming DA, Edison KE, Pak H. Telehealth ethics. Telemed J E Health. 2009;15(8):797–803. https://doi.org/10.1089/tmj.2009.0035.
30. Chaet D, Clearfield R, Sabin JE, Skimming K, Council on Ethical and Judicial Affairs American Medical Association. Ethical practice in telehealth and telemedicine. J Gen Intern Med. 2017;32(10):1136–40. https://doi.org/10.1007/s11606-017-4082-2.
31. Sax M. Privacy from an ethical perspective. In: Van der Sloot B, De Groot A, editors. The handbook of privacy studies: an interdisciplinary introduction. Amsterdam: Amsterdam University Press. p. 143–73.
32. Government of Canada Interagency Advisory Panel on Research Ethics. TCPS 2. Chapter 5: privacy and confidentiality. 2022. https://ethics.gc.ca/eng/tcps2-eptc2_2022_chapter5-chapitre5.html#intro. Accessed 18 Apr 2024.
33. Wright AJ. Tele-health and clinical assessment (tele-assessment). In: Encyclopedia of mental health, vol. 1–3. 3rd ed. Elsevier; 2023. p. V3-418–V3-25.
34. Nittari G, Khuman R, Baldoni S, Pallotta G, Battineni G, Sirignano A, et al. Telemedicine practice: review of the current ethical and legal challenges. Telemed J E Health. 2020;26(12):1427–37. https://doi.org/10.1089/tmj.2019.0158.

Ethics in Telerehabilitation

12

Hatice Adiguzel Tat

12.1 Telerehabilitation

Telehealth encompasses a wide range of modalities, encompassing both clinical and nonclinical services. Telerehabilitation can be considered as a subset of telemedicine, which has seen a surge in adoption thanks to advancements in computer science technologies and telemedical devices. Telerehabilitation refers specifically to clinical rehabilitation services with the focus of evaluation, diagnosis, and treatment [1, 2]. To shorten hospital stays for patients and save money for both patients and healthcare providers, telerehabilitation has been developed to care for inpatients and discharge them following the acute phase of an illness [1, 3]. Through telerehabilitation, the traditional face-to-face method of patient-rehabilitator interaction can be replaced, allowing for the treatment of acute phases of disorders [1, 3]. There exist reports on the range of telerehabilitation treatment modalities, as well as their corresponding lengths and intensities. Telerehabilitation can manifest in various forms, including asynchronous e-visits, virtual check-ins, two-way real-time visits utilizing audio, video, or both, remote evaluations of recorded videos or photos, and assessments conducted via telephone. Even before the pandemic, the Department of Veterans Affairs was a pioneer in the field of telerehabilitation, with a sharp increase in the usage of remote services, such as physical therapy [4]. Until the demands for safer service delivery spurred by COVID-19, the widespread adoption of telerehabilitation across various health systems and throughout the country has been hindered by inconsistencies and restrictions in state regulations, Medicare reimbursement policies, and the rules set by private insurers [5].

H. Adiguzel Tat (✉)
Department of Physiotherapy and Rehabilitation, Faculty of Health Sciences, Kahramanmaras Sutcu Imam University, Onikisubat, Turkey
e-mail: haticadiguzel@ksu.edu.tr

F. Özden et al. (eds.), *Telerehabilitation*, TELe-Health,
https://doi.org/10.1007/978-3-031-69080-8_12

The utilization of telerehabilitation for physical therapy is now permitted under recent changes in laws and regulations, offering previously unheard-of research opportunities regarding the applications and outcomes of telerehabilitation [2]. According to several systematic reviews, telerehabilitation proves advantageous for individuals dealing with musculoskeletal disorders, multiple sclerosis, osteoarthritis, and deficits in motor function [6–8]. Telerehabilitation can also lower medical expenses, increase treatment compliance, enhance quality of life, and enhance both mental and physical function when provided to patients in a way that meets their needs [2, 9, 10]. The results of synchronous, real-time rehabilitation are the focus of the majority of telerehabilitation research, yet there is some indication that asynchronous telemedicine may also be beneficial for some patient populations, such as those who have had total joint replacement. However, more research is required to answer concerns regarding the viability, security, and efficacy of telerehabilitation modalities in various patient demographics and environments, including those with frailty or at risk of fall [2, 11].

In order to understand the scope and application of telerehabilitation, as well as to determine the duration, types, recipients, and ethical principles of telerehabilitation, it is essential to conduct research on similar practices in the real world. Descriptive studies can be carried out by researchers utilizing "administrative and claims data" to investigate the effects of policy changes on the provision of rehabilitation and telerehabilitation modalities. Researchers can, for instance, look at how telerehabilitation codes were used prior to the pandemic and monitor changes in that usage following the publication of Centers for Medicare & Medicaid Services waivers authorizing telerehabilitation [2]. To promote changes and address disparities, data scientists working with clinical data inside a health system can produce real-time reports on practice. Utilizing already-existing data, such as Medicare claims data or electronic health record data, is an essential first step in estimating the impact of policy on implementation, provider utilization, and patient outcomes with regard to telerehabilitation [2]. Descriptive studies of this nature, employing standardized data elements to code care delivery, health status, and outcomes—including functional outcomes, as well as critical indicators like hospital readmissions and injurious falls—require a comprehensive grasp of the continuously evolving federal and state regulations governing practice and reimbursement [2]. Research on the delivery of outpatient physiotherapy within healthcare systems, employing standardized patient-reported outcome measures, can facilitate comparisons between specific patient subgroups (such as individuals with particular diagnoses or conditions) receiving standard care and those undergoing telerehabilitation [2].

12.2 Ethics in Telerehabilitation

The World Medical Association defines ethics as "the study of morality, involving deliberate and systematic reflection and analysis of moral decisions and behaviors, whether past, present, or future" [12]. Since ethics is applied in situations when the law permits freedom of choice, it is a complicated concept. The World Health

Organization (WHO) recommends individual autonomy, beneficence, non-maleficence, and the equitable sharing of benefits and limits as ethical principles [12]. Concerns about privacy, patient autonomy, universal accessibility, and professional secrecy are among the ethical considerations surrounding the development of telerehabilitation [13]. Both reminding practitioners of the ethical framework that governs medical practice and supplying information to stakeholders can promote the ethical growth of telerehabilitation [13]. In projects developing telerehabilitation guidelines, ethical considerations are often glossed over and without explanation. Hence, it became essential to examine the ethical considerations raised by telerehabilitation and to devise solutions to address these concerns. This is crucial for guiding telerehabilitation programs toward ethical practices in these areas [13]. The three most important ethical guidelines for telerehabilitation are accountability for covering potential losses from the therapist or treatment facility, professional commitment, and privacy and security [14]. All of the requirements for face-to-face rehabilitation should be satisfied when providing telerehabilitation services. One of the primary barriers to the broad application of telerehabilitation is the absence of global ethical standards in this field. The ethical standards in this domain need to be well-defined, and telerehabilitation technologies need to meet certain requirements in order to apply this strategy correctly and successfully [14].

Organizations regulate the operational aspects of healthcare institutions through their own policies and procedures. Since the introduction of telemedicine, there has been an increasing tendency to provide telehealth services without properly examining the moral and legal ramifications [15]. Potential applications of digital and electronic services in telerehabilitation may have an impact on a number of moral and legal considerations, including carelessness, permission, and secrecy. It is therefore essential to develop precise tactics in this regard. State laws, cultural norms, and religious beliefs all have an impact on the ethical and legal aspects of healthcare [15].

Analyzing the delivery of telerehabilitation over time and in different geographic regions can show whether and how the pandemic, stay-at-home orders, and broadband or Internet availability affect utilization differently by patients and providers at the system level [2]. Analyses at the patient level are able to spot unintentional delays or disturbances in care as well as investigate patient experiences, such as contentment with, trust in, and perception of the acceptability of technology for medical treatment and interaction with the medical staff [2].

Treatment outcomes using telerehabilitation probably differ depending on the severity and condition of the patient. The possibility of a sizable quantity of unmeasured confounding and possibly missing data is inherent in observational research because of the difficulties in providing care during COVID-19 [2]. These kinds of research will need to look at prevalent patient problems and use the right analytical techniques to account for comorbidities, severity, and other factors influencing patient care. These techniques include imputation for missing data, controls for selection bias (like using instrumental variables and the inverse probability of treatment weighting), risk adjustment techniques (like using propensity scores and controlling for potential confounders in models), and other techniques frequently used in health services research [16, 17]. Preliminary studies with adequately sized samples will initiate the identification of patient subgroups that may benefit or not from certain telerehabilitation techniques. When making decisions regarding whether to continue offering telerehabilitation services, these statistics will be crucial. If there is sufficient planning to address equipoise in care delivery, capacity for research in practice during or after the pandemic, and appropriate methodological expertise available, more rigorous study designs such as pragmatic trials and hybrid implementation-effectiveness studies should be considered. In the end, if telerehabilitation therapies can demonstrate outcomes that are comparable to or more cost-effective than conventional care, there would be compelling evidence to support the continued integration of telerehabilitation as a care delivery option even after the pandemic subsides [2].

Despite being relatively new, telerehabilitation is becoming increasingly popular in industrialized nations. Telerehabilitation is generally less expensive for patients and healthcare providers than traditional inpatient or person-to-person rehabilitation [1]. Moreover, this technology could offer assistance to patients in rural areas where traditional rehabilitation programs may not be easily accessible. Nevertheless, it's crucial to acknowledge some drawbacks of telerehabilitation, including patients' potential mistrust stemming from virtual communication with their doctors or rehabilitation professionals [1]. Thus, it can be beneficial for health personnel and patients to get to know each other, for satisfaction, cooperation, and trust. Furthermore, this collaboration requires informed consent from all patients. Although telerehabilitation is a relatively new and intriguing field, there are currently no established protocols or standard operating procedures, and many telerehabilitation facilities are only being used for pilot projects [1].

Ensuring patient privacy necessitates the adoption of telerehabilitation procedures within the framework of ethical norms. A primary barrier to the successful and widespread adoption of these techniques is the lack of international standards regarding the ethics of telerehabilitation and the absence of pertinent legislative provisions [18]. There are millions of definitions for ethics, which may be the most significant problem in telehealth. As telemedicine advances, new moral and legal dilemmas surface [18].

In order to use telerehabilitation in a way that respects ethical standards, it is necessary for various players to engage in ethical reflection in order for them to be aware of the concerns and the program's underlying points of vigilance. Therefore, in a telerehabilitation program, all actors will be stimulated. Thus, there are three levels at which the ethical framework could be used. First, the quality of communication needs to be given considerably greater consideration. This is presuming that health professionals had attended training sessions where they were taught about communication tools, the connection between motivation and practice, and the consequences of using such a tool. It is crucial that physiotherapists receive training on digital health [19].

12.2.1 Electronic Medical Record Systems and Ethics

Better and faster patient data sharing between and within the institution, data access when needed, improved data protection, and an increase in accuracy can all be achieved with the help of an electronic medical record (EMR), which will improve medical decision-making and reduce the risk of adverse drug reactions [18, 20]. Certain protected circumstances and ethical guidelines must be followed in EMR systems. Possible risks of copying and pasting data from other providers for any reason is one of these issues. Possible risks include the security of personal data, the accuracy or timeliness of copied information, as well as the illegal transfer of personal data to other databases. These confusions may also be due to the staff's doubts about clinical data in some EMRs and incomplete data entry after the deadline [18, 21, 22]. The template data that software provides to make therapists' jobs easier is one of the most prevalent ethical issues. Patient-specific data are entered into these templates and recorded. Inaccurate patient evaluation records into the system arise from improper use of these templates. Clinicians should exercise caution while utilizing these comparable software shortcuts [21, 22]. The fact that EMRs are not used for patient document recording and storage, but rather for billing and storing proof data for health insurance, is one of the most prevalent ethical issues. When only billing features of the software are used, pathology codes are only used for price purposes, and other similar uses, the efficiency of EMRs is decreased [23]. For the right safety of patient data, it's critical to manage technological elements including intrusive attacks, firewalls, antivirus programs, and software updates [24].

Ethical concerns such as informed consent, privacy, security, and social media norms are highlighted in recent publications by the American Counseling Association (ACA, 2014), the Commission on Rehabilitation Counselor Certification (2017), and the National Board for Certified Counselors (NBCC, 2016a). Using an ethical decision-making model, obtaining training, establishing clear limits with clients through an informed consent approach, and obtaining compliant software are some suggestions for practitioners to handle ethical difficulties [25]. Below are some ideas for safeguarding patients' ethical components in online and mobile applications created for patients undergoing telerehabilitation who are evaluated and treated remotely [25].

***Informed Consent*:** Since technology is used so widely, electronic consent forms that are given to patients should mitigate any potential ethical transgressions. An informed permission form that covers legal guidelines, privacy concerns, possible danger scenarios, and the benefits and drawbacks of telerehabilitation with regard to software technology use should be signed by patients [26].

***Patient Access to Telerehabilitation*:** Despite recent increases in Internet infrastructure and electronic communication equipment, many populations, particularly those living in rural areas, may not have enough of these resources given their socioeconomic status. The potential infrastructure needed to provide significant volumes of data to the patient population in this group might not be suitable, even if the facilities are adequate. It is morally required that we not stop these patients from utilizing mHealth (mobile phone technologies-Health) [27].

Identity Verification, Data Ownership, and Hacking by Third Parties: There is never an assurance regarding the security of the data gathered via telerehabilitation. Hackers and third-party apps produce medical data that results in large financial losses. Authentication techniques like "two factor authentication" have been created to safeguard this. Modern encryption techniques still fall short of providing the appropriate level of protection for such data [28].

Privacy and Security: One of the most crucial ethical precepts is safeguarding patient confidentiality and privacy when using software for telerehabilitation systems. Measures should be taken to reduce the possibility of inappropriate disclosure of information in these databases, including patient personal data. User agreements should be developed within the parameters of ethical and legal requirements in order to safeguard the privacy of patient information [29].

The three most crucial telerehabilitation ethics standards are patient consent, software security, and personal data protection [18].

12.3 Guidelines of Different Countries in Telerehabilitation

12.3.1 The Principles of the American Telemedical Association for Providing Telerehabilitation Services

The American Telemedicine Association's (ATA) "A Blueprint for Telerehabilitation Guidelines" (2010) elucidates definitions and the scope of telerehabilitation, establishes administrative principles including informed consent and considerations for billing and coding under different reimbursement models, enhances clinical principles, and revises technical standards [30]. This document's content focuses on general administrative, clinical, technical, and ethical concepts rather than offering detailed implementation practice guidelines for telerehabilitation services. This manual is not meant to take the place of a primary practitioner's clinical judgment when determining the best course of treatment for a particular patient. The ATA's document recognizes that professional development and training may be essential to foster effective delivery of rehabilitation and habilitation services via information and communication technology (ICT), as well as to uphold best practice standards [30].

12.3.1.1 ATA's Administrative Principles

- Alongside other credentialing, privileging, accrediting, and regulatory prerequisites for licensing, certification, professional liability, and ongoing professional development or training related to the use of communication telerehabilitation systems for delivering provisional services and products, organizations and professionals must remain cognizant of and adhere to the laws, regulations, guidelines, and standards established by nationally recognized professional associations [30].
- Professionals and/or organizations must be aware of and abide by all applicable federal, state, and local laws and licensure requirements [30].

- When introducing telerehabilitation services, organizations and professionals must also consider and adhere to any additional operational or contractual requirements or arrangements that may be necessary or vital [30].
- Professional rules, organization policies regarding informed consent, and federal and state telehealth laws must all be known to and followed by organizations and/or professionals. During a virtual encounter, the client is informed and educated about the extent of the telerehabilitation services through the informed consent, which covers topics such as service types, technology used, recording of audio, video, and/or photo content, use of support staff, record-keeping, privacy and security, ending services, payment plans, and other encounter-related details [30].
- All relevant forms of licensure portability (such as expedited licenses, limited licenses, and Interstate Licensure Compacts) that may have an impact on interstate practice must be known by organizations and professionals [30].
- Professionals and organizations must have a system in place to make sure that customers are informed about their rights and obligations when it comes to using telerehabilitation services and/or their personal health records, as well as how to file complaints and grievances [30].
- When delivering telerehabilitation services, organizations and/or professionals must be mindful of and adhere to the latest privacy, security, and confidentiality regulations [30].
- Professionals, organizations, and commercial insurers need to stay informed about the latest billing and coding procedures, including the application of designated modifiers or specific codes as mandated by state or federal insurance plans, commercial insurers, or private health plan payment policies. It is essential for providers to have a thorough understanding of the various reimbursement arrangements, agreements, and alternative payment methodologies currently in place. These may encompass fee-for-services, bundled care, accountable care organizations, primary care medical homes, shared savings, partial risk, and other payment models incorporating cost savings and avoidance metrics [30].
- To cater to the needs of clients before, during, and after telerehabilitation sessions, organizations and professionals must ensure the availability of a suitable facilitator, telepresenter, translator, or e-helper. This individual could be a caregiver, family member, provider, or another authorized person [30].
- To ensure the client's safety in case of a health-related complication, organizations and professionals should consider implementing mechanisms, policies, and procedures to verify the client's location during virtual encounters, establish backup modes of communication (such as text or phone), and develop an emergency plan [30].
- Participants in study procedures must be protected, according to organizations and experts involved in telerehabilitation research. In order to facilitate participant decision-making and informed consent, research protocols must be authorized by the linked agency's research/ethical review body (such as the Institutional Review Board) and adhere to all applicable laws and regulations [30].

12.3.1.2 ATA's Clinical Principles

Professionals must integrate the guidelines and standards established by nationally recognized professional associations into their practices. This should be done in conjunction with fulfilling other requirements such as credentialing, privileging, accrediting, and regulatory obligations for licensing, certification, professional liability, and ongoing professional development or training to provide temporary services and products. Additionally, they must be knowledgeable about and adhere to laws and regulations, as well as stay informed about and comply with all guidelines for scope of practice policies and the requirements of professional state boards [30]. Professionals who supply information or services using hardware, software, or devices should be trained in the operation and troubleshooting of equipment and software, or they should always have access to technology vendors and support to help with technical issues. Moreover, to effectively integrate and adapt any instructions, interventions, materials, or accessories used during an encounter, providers should possess proficiency in utilizing videoconferencing accessories, including data exchange tools [30]. To cater to the needs of both the client and the provider before, during, and after the telerehabilitation session, professionals must ensure the availability of an appropriate facilitator, telepresenter, translator, or e-helper (which could be a caregiver, family member, provider, or another authorized individual) as needed [30]. When delivering synchronous (real-time interactive) or asynchronous (store-and-forward) telerehabilitation services, professionals must consider the need to adapt educational or intervention materials, methods, tools, and/or the physical environment accordingly [30].

12.3.1.3 ATA's Technical Principles

At the time of clinical interactions, organizations and professionals are responsible for making sure that the equipment is safe, adequate, and operating as intended to support diagnostic and/or treatment needs. This involves keeping extra gadgets or auxiliary technologies (such as measuring equipment, sound meters, sensor technologies, etc.) on hand in case they are needed for assessments and treatments [30]. Professionals and organizations must abide by all applicable laws, rules, and codes pertaining to technology and technological safety. Infection control policies and procedures that adhere to organizational, national, state, and local regulatory standards for the use of telehealth equipment and peripherals must be in place for organizations and professionals. Mechanisms must be in place to specifically clean and sterilize equipment so that it can be reused by multiple customers [30].

12.3.1.4 ATA's Ethical Principles

Policies that identify, eliminate, and lessen conflicts of interest related to the provision of telerehabilitation services should also be in place within organizations and among experts. When obtaining rehabilitation and habilitation services through telerehabilitation, professionals are required to advise clients of their rights and duties, including the ability to decline or stop receiving services [30, 31]. Also professionals are expected to integrate organizational ethics and values into telerehabilitation policies and processes. And they must follow professional codes of ethics and be aware of and abide by all applicable laws, rules, legislation, and/or policies pertaining to telerehabilitation [30, 31].

References

1. Peretti A, Amenta F, Tayebati SK, Nittari G, Mahdi SS. Tele-rehabilitation: review of the state-of-the-art and areas of application. JMIR Rehabil Assist Technol. 2017;4(2):e7511.
2. Prvu Bettger J, Resnik LJ. Tele-rehabilitation in the age of COVID-19: an opportunity for learning health system research. Phys Ther. 2020;100(11):1913–6.
3. Carey JR, Durfee WK, Bhatt E, Nagpal A, Weinstein SA, Anderson KM, et al. Comparison of finger tracking versus simple movement training via tele-rehabilitation to alter hand function and cortical reorganization after stroke. Neurorehabil Neural Repair. 2007;21(3):216–32.
4. Cowper-Ripley DC, Jia H, Wang X, Freytes IM, Hale-Gallardo J, Castaneda G, et al. Trends in VA tele-rehabilitation patients and encounters over time and by rurality. Fed Pract. 2019;36(3):122.
5. Bierman RT, Kwong MW, Calouro C. State occupational and physical therapy telehealth laws and regulations: a 50-state survey. Int J Telerehabil. 2018;10(2):3.
6. Agostini M, Moja L, Banzi R, Pistotti V, Tonin P, Venneri A, et al. Tele-rehabilitation and recovery of motor function: a systematic review and meta-analysis. J Telemed Telecare. 2015;21(4):202–13.
7. Cottrell MA, Galea OA, O'Leary SP, Hill AJ, Russell TG. Real-time tele-rehabilitation for the treatment of musculoskeletal conditions is effective and comparable to standard practice: a systematic review and meta-analysis. Clin Rehabil. 2017;31(5):625–38.
8. Grona SL, Bath B, Busch A, Rotter T, Trask C, Harrison E. Use of videoconferencing for physical therapy in people with musculoskeletal conditions: a systematic review. J Telemed Telecare. 2018;24(5):341–55.
9. Bettger JP, Green CL, Holmes DN, Chokshi A, Mather RC III, Hoch BT, et al. Effects of virtual exercise rehabilitation in-home therapy compared with traditional care after total knee arthroplasty: VERITAS, a randomized controlled trial. JBJS. 2020;102(2):101–9.
10. Tousignant M, Boissy P, Corriveau H, Moffet H. In home Tele-rehabilitation for older adults after discharge from an acute hospital or rehabilitation unit: a proof-of-concept study and costs estimation. Disabil Rehabil Assist Technol. 2006;1(4):209–16.
11. Bini S, Mahajan J. Clinical outcomes of remote asynchronous Tele-rehabilitation are equivalent to traditional therapy following total knee arthroplasty: a randomized control study. J Telemed Telecare. 2017;23(2):239–47.
12. World Health Organization. Comités d'éthique de la recherche: notions de base pour le renforcement des capacités. WHO; 2009.
13. Guy M, Blary A, Ladner J, Gilliaux M. Ethical issues linked to the development of telerehabilitation: a qualitative study. Int J Telerehabil. 2021;13(1):e6367.
14. Babazadeh Zavieh SS, Haeri SMJ, Shariat A. Ethical principles in tele-rehabilitation: a narrative review. Islamic Life J. 2023;7(1):110–6.
15. Alhabter AM, Qureshi AZ, Ullah S. Ethical and legal aspects of tele-rehabilitation in Saudi Arabia. Int J Telerehabil. 2023;15(2):e6569.
16. Seaman SR, White IR. Review of inverse probability weighting for dealing with missing data. Stat Methods Med Res. 2013;22(3):278–95.
17. Stoto M, Oakes M, Stuart E, Brown R, Zurovac J, Priest EL. Analytical methods for a learning health system: 3. analysis of observational studies. eGEMs. 2017;5(1):30.
18. Ozden F, Lembarki Y. The ethical necessities and principles in tele-rehabilitation. Sağlık Hizmetleri ve Eğitimi Dergisi. 2020;3(2):35–7.

19. Brennan D, Tindall L, Theodoros D, Brown J, Campbell M, Christiana D, et al. A blueprint for tele-rehabilitation guidelines. Int J Telerehabil. 2010;2(2):31.
20. Clifford GD, Blaya JA, Hall-Clifford R, Fraser HS. Medical information systems: a foundation for healthcare technologies in developing countries. Springer; 2008.
21. Hammond KW, Helbig ST, Benson CC, Brathwaite-Sketoe BM, editors. Are electronic medical records trustworthy? Observations on copying, pasting and duplication. AMIA Annual Symposium Proceedings. American Medical Informatics Association; 2003.
22. Menachemi N, Collum TH. Benefits and drawbacks of electronic health record systems. Risk Manag Healthc Policy. 2011;4:47–55.
23. Bernat JL. Ethical and quality pitfalls in electronic health records. Neurology. 2013;80(11):1057–61.
24. Chiuchisan I, Balan D-G, Geman O, Chiuchisan I, Gordin I, editors. A security approach for health care information systems. 2017 E-health and bioengineering conference (EHB). IEEE; 2017.
25. Holmes CM, Reid CA. Ethics in tele-rehabilitation: looking ahead. J Appl Rehabil Couns. 2018;49(2):14–23.
26. Recupero PR, Rainey SE. Informed consent to e-therapy. Am J Psychother. 2005;59(4):319–31.
27. Carter A, Liddle J, Hall W, Chenery H. Mobile phones in research and treatment: ethical guidelines and future directions. JMIR Mhealth Uhealth. 2015;3(4):e4538.
28. He D, Naveed M, Gunter CA, Nahrstedt K, editors. Security concerns in Android mHealth apps. AMIA annual symposium proceedings. American Medical Informatics Association; 2014.
29. Stanberry B. Legal ethical and risk issues in telemedicine. Comput Methods Prog Biomed. 2001;64(3):225–33.
30. Richmond T, Peterson C, Cason J, Billings M, Terrell EA, Lee ACW, et al. American Telemedicine Association's principles for delivering tele-rehabilitation services. Int J Telerehabil. 2017;9(2):63.
31. Sarsak HI. Tele-rehabilitation services: a successful paradigm for occupational therapy clinical services. Int Phys Med Rehabil J. 2020;5(2):93–8.

MIX
Papier aus verantwortungsvollen Quellen
Paper from responsible sources
FSC® C105338

FSC
www.fsc.org

If you have any concerns about our products,
you can contact us on
ProductSafety@springernature.com

In case Publisher is established outside the EU,
the EU authorized representative is:
Springer Nature Customer Service Center GmbH
Europaplatz 3, 69115 Heidelberg, Germany

Printed by Libri Plureos GmbH
in Hamburg, Germany